THE MIND COOKBOOK

Quick and Delicious Recipes for Enhancing Brain Function and Helping Prevent Alzheimer's and Dementia

KRISTIN DIVERSI

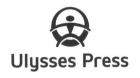

Ulysses Press

Published in the United States by:
ULYSSES PRESS
P.O. Box 3440
Berkeley, CA 94703
www.ulyssespress.com

ISBN: 978-1-61243-725-5
Library of Congress Control Number: 2017938174

Printed in Canada by Marquis Book Printing
10 9 8 7 6 5 4 3 2 1

Acquisitions editor: Bridget Thoreson
Managing editor: Claire Chun
Project editor: Alice Riegert
Editor: Shayna Keyles
Proofreader: Nancy Bell
Production: Caety Klingman, Jake Flaherty
Front cover design: Rebecca Lown
Cover photos from shutterstock.com: salmon © Jacek Chabraszewski;
    blueberries © Elena Schweitzer; chicken © Barbara Dudzinska;
    pumpkin soup © allstars; nuts © Ilja Generalov

Distributed by Publishers Group West

NOTE TO READERS: This book has been written and published strictly for informational and educational purposes only. It is not intended to serve as medical advice or to be any form of medical treatment. You should always consult your physician before altering or changing any aspect of your medical treatment and/or undertaking a diet regimen, including the guidelines as described in this book. Do not stop or change any prescription medications without the guidance and advice of your physician. Any use of the information in this book is made on the reader's good judgment after consulting with his or her physician and is the reader's sole responsibility. This book is not intended to diagnose or treat any medical condition and is not a substitute for a physician.

This book is independently authored and published and no sponsorship or endorsement of this book by, and no affiliation with, any trademarked brands or other products mentioned within is claimed or suggested. All trademarks that appear in ingredient lists and elsewhere in this book belong to their respective owners and are used here for informational purposes only. The author and publisher encourage readers to patronize the quality brands mentioned and pictured in this book.

For marigolds and apple pie
And a red sun hat
Dedicated to a Force of a woman,
My Nanny,
Shirley Douglas.

CONTENTS

THE AGING BRAIN AND WHAT YOU CAN DO

As we age, our brains, like our bodies, go through many changes. These changes are influenced by several factors like genetics, neurotransmitters (the chemicals in our brain that send messages), hormones, and life experiences.[1] Research has identified that the main factors that increase the risk of diseases such as Alzheimer's and dementia are age, family history, and heredity. While we can't change those influencers, we can make transformations to our lifestyles to reduce the effects of brain-aging.[2]

The greatest risk factors for brain-aging related conditions like Alzheimer's disease and dementia are:

- Being aged 65 or older
- Having one or more close family member with the diseases
- Having a genetic predisposition for the diseases

The majority of brain-aging related diseases, however, occur from a complex interaction of factors. Even without brain-aging related diseases, the brain does age as our bodies do. We often see changes in size and volume, vasculature (or arrangement/

---

1   Ruth Peters, "Ageing and the Brain," *Postgraduate Medical Journal* 82, no. 964 (Feb 2006): 84–88, doi: 10.1136/pgmj.2005.036665.
2   Alzheimer's Association, "Risk Factors," accessed Jul 23, 2017, http://www.alz.org/alzheimers_disease_causes_risk_factors.asp.

network of blood vessels), and cognition as we get older. Our brains naturally shrink in volume, particularly in the frontal cortex (responsible for attention, memory, learning new information, and creativity[3]), as we age.[4]

With rising blood pressure and aging blood vessels our vasculature can destabilize, increasing the risk of stroke. Due to these factors, we often develop ischemia, or inadequate blood supply, to areas of our bodies, like the brain. Even relatively healthy people may develop lesions on their white matter (the signaling part of the brain) as they age, which may influence our mental and physical function and even lead to diseases and disorders like dementia and multiple sclerosis, among others.[5]

But there is good news! There are simple, protective actions you can take to mitigate the changes of an aging brain. Research shows that healthy lifestyle practices, like regular exercise, cognitive exercises, and, finally, a healthy diet can help prevent, slow, and even halt the changes of an aging brain.[6] This book is based on a diet that was designed with an aging brain in mind. No matter if you are at risk for Alzheimer's or dementia or you just want to take the first step to a healthier brain, this book is for you. With recipes that follow the MIND Diet, you will be on the road to protecting and maintaining the health of your brain in no time.

---

3   S.V. Siddiqui, et. al., "Neuropsychology of prefrontal cortex," *Indian Journal of Psychiatry* 50, no. 3 (Jul 2008): 202–8, doi: 10.4103/0019-5545.43634.

4   Ibid.

5   K.W. Kim, et. al., "Classification of white matter lesions on magnetic resonance imaging in elderly persons," *Biological Psychiatry* 64, no. 4 (Aug 2008): 273–80, doi: 10.1016/j.biopsych.2008.03.024.

6   Peters, "Ageing and the Brain," *Postgraduate Medical Journal*, 84–88.

What Is the MIND Diet?

A well-balanced diet is the foundation to general health, but what if it were the foundation to brain health, as well? The MIND Diet is the first diet specifically geared toward promoting not just better health in general, but better brain health throughout life.

Revolutionized by nutritional epidemiology expert, Dr. Martha Clare Morris, in 2015, the MIND Diet is a combination of two existing diets, the Mediterranean Diet and the DASH Diet. The Mediterranean Diet is based on the dietary habits of the populations of Greece, Southern Italy, and Spain. It has gained popularity in recent years for focusing on fresh, whole foods; using healthy fats; and promoting the health benefits of wine. Research suggests that the Mediterranean Diet has protective properties against cardiovascular disease, diabetes, and cancer, and it has been linked to living a longer life overall. Some research also supports links to brain health, including reducing the risk of Alzheimer's disease, possibly owing to its focus on antioxidant foods and those that reduce inflammation.[7]

Developed by the National Institutes of Health, the DASH Diet was created to prevent and control hypertension without the use of medication. The diet focuses on fruits and vegetables, low-fat dairy, whole grains, lean meats, nuts, and beans. Research reports that the diet significantly reduces blood pressure for those with even moderate hypertension, which is a risk factor for Alzheimer's disease. Lowering blood pressure through diet may be a preventative factor for Alzheimer's disease. Like the Mediterranean Diet, the DASH Diet is only beginning to be studied for effects on brain health, but one study of 800 senior citizens from the Memory and

---

7 "MIND Diet," *U.S. News*, accessed Feb 7, 2017, http://health.usnews.com/best-diet/mind-diet.

Aging Project found an association between compliance with the diet with lower rates of cognitive decline.[8]

The MIND Diet distinguishes itself from these two diets in that it is less demanding than either. It doesn't require as many servings of fish, grains, fruits, or vegetables, and there's no emphasis on dairy or limits on total fat. It's also different in that the MIND Diet specifically recommends leafy green vegetables and berries above other types of vegetables and fruit—although other fruits and vegetables are still recommended.

The MIND Diet was created by Dr. Morris, after reviewing the existing literature surrounding brain health and food, specifically examining the Mediterranean Diet and the DASH Diet. She then conducted a study to test the effects of a combination of these diets on nearly 1,000 senior citizens in the Chicago area of the United States, aged 58 to 98, for an average of four and a half years. Using a guided questionnaire, diets were assessed based on how closely they matched up to the Mediterranean, DASH, and MIND Diets, and the cognitive function of participants was measured every year using 19 different cognitive tests. The study showed that the MIND Diet, when observed moderately well, lowered the risk of Alzheimer's by approximately 35 percent and by 53 percent when observed rigorously.[9]

However, Dr. Morris reminds us that "there appear to be many factors that play into who gets the disease, including behavioral, environmental, and genetic components."[10]

---

8   Ibid.

9   Ibid.

10   Nancy Di Fiore, "Diet May Help Prevent Alzheimer's," Rush University Medical Center, accessed Jul 15, 2017, https://www.rush.edu/news/diet-may-help-prevent-alzheimers.

AN INTRODUCTION TO ALZHEIMER'S DISEASE AND DEMENTIA

Dementia and Alzheimer's disease are not the same thing, although many people think that they are and may even swap out the terms. Alzheimer's disease is actually the most common cause of dementia. People who develop Alzheimer's disease may experience symptoms such as confusion, becoming lost in previously familiar places and settings, or difficulty with tasks and with language, such as trouble remembering the right words. Dementia is a condition that causes a person to have difficulties with "normal" cognitive functions, like making judgments, applying reasoning, or using memory.

Alzheimer's disease is progressive, and it affects the nerve cells in the parts of the brain that are mainly responsible for memory, cognition, language, and motor skills. Science hasn't yet found a genetic cause for Alzheimer's disease. For now, we focus on environmental factors that may play a role in its development.[11] The current pharmaceutical treatments approved by the FDA only treat the symptoms of Alzheimer's, and that is temporary relief, at best. These are not effective cures.[12] Alzheimer's disease can begin to develop ten to twenty years before a person even notices its symptoms. By the time people with Alzheimer's disease, or their families, notice any changes in memory or other cognitive differences, they may be in mild or late stage Alzheimer's, and the damage to their brain is already progressing.

---

11   Nancy Bartolotti and Orly Lazarov, "Lifestyle and Alzheimer's Disease: The Role of Environmental Factors in Disease Development," *Genes, Environment, and Alzheimer's Disease* (2016): 197–237, doi: 10.1016/B978-0-12-802851-3.00007-3.

12   Christina Dailey, "The Impact of Alzheimer's Disease—The Silent Killer," *JCCC Honors Journal* 7, no. 2 (Spring 2016): 1–14, http://scholarspace.jccc.edu/cgi/viewcontent.cgi?article=1064&context=honors_journal.

There are currently no treatments for stopping or reversing this damage, which is why prevention is the best way that we know of to treat Alzheimer's disease. Focusing on prevention factors could reduce the risk of Alzheimer's disease by as much as 25 to 45 percent. It will also reduce the risk of other diseases that are correlated with Alzheimer's disease and dementia, such as heart disease, hypertension, Type 2 diabetes, obesity, and depression.[13] Alzheimer's disease costs the United States alone over $200 billion dollars every year. By 2050, it is estimated that one out of 85 people worldwide will suffer from Alzheimer's disease.[14]

The good news is that, contrary to popular belief, the effects of an aging brain are not inevitable. Some research suggests that certain lifestyle factors may help delay symptoms associated with Alzheimer's disease and dementia. These include finding meaning in your life or work, keeping a network of friends and family, exercising regularly, keeping your brain active and engaged in motivating activities, and eating a diet that is rich in omega-3 fatty acids, vegetables, and olive oil. That's where the MIND Diet comes in. While diets that are high in saturated, unhealthy fats and cholesterol have been linked to cognitive decline, research is showing that diets rich in omega-3 fatty acids help reduce the risk not only of Alzheimer's disease and dementia, but of the diseases correlated with dementia, mentioned above. As with any medical condition, the best person to speak with if you have any concerns for yourself or your loved one will be your doctor.[15]

---

13   Ibid.
14   Ibid.
15   Rush University Alzheimer's Disease Center, accessed Feb 2017, https://www.rush.edu/services/conditions/alzheimers-disease.

What Makes the MIND Diet Successful?

The foods chosen for the MIND Diet are rich in antioxidants and anti-inflammatory properties.

Nutrients like flavonoids, carotenoids, vitamin E, omega-3 fatty acids, folate, and vitamins C and D,[16] have been shown to slow cognitive decline and help neurons cope with the stress related to aging. These nutrients help repair damage to the brain, protect it from new harm, and make it more difficult for new injury to occur.

The MIND Diet hones all the best aspects from the Mediterranean and the DASH diets, emphasizing the best foods for brain health—targeting ten specific brain-healthy food groups and asking participants to avoid just five. Plus, the MIND Diet is not nearly as strict as the Mediterranean or DASH diets.

Foods to Enjoy

On the MIND Diet, participants are encouraged to focus on eating primarily from the following ten food groups:

GREEN LEAFY VEGETABLES: Some common examples of green, leafy vegetables you'll find in this book are arugula, spinach, and kale. Loaded with brain-healthy nutrients like folate, vitamin E, and flavonoids, the MIND Diet suggests that you get at least one serving per day.

Servings: 1 serving per day, at least

Serving size: 2 cups raw leafy greens or 1 cup cooked leafy greens

---

16   Judith C. Thalheimer, "The MIND Diet—Fighting Dementia with Food," *Today's Geriatric Medicine* 8, no. 4 (Jul/Aug 2015): 10, accessed Jul 15, 2017, http://www.todaysgeriatricmedicine.com/archive/0715p10.shtml.

SERVING SIZE ESTIMATIONS

1 cup = your fist

1 ounce = the meaty part of your thumb

1 tablespoon = your thumb, minus the meaty part

1 teaspoon = the tip of your index finger

1 to 2 ounces of a food like nuts = your cupped hand

3 ounces of meat, fish, or poultry = the palm of your hand

BERRIES: High in flavonoids, berries have been shown to improve short- and long-term cognition. In this book, we'll explores recipes with blueberries, raspberries, strawberries and more. Did you know that bananas are a type of berry? They are! The MIND Diet suggests at least two servings per week of berries.

Servings: 2 servings per week, at least

Serving size: 1 cup fresh fruit or ½ cup dried fruit

VEGETABLES AND FRUIT: The MIND Diet recommends at least one serving per day of vegetables and fruits, like broccoli, sweet potato, or apples, all of which we'll work with in this book. Full of vitamins like folate and vitamin B6, vegetable intake is associated with improved cognitive function.

Servings: 1 serving per day, at least

Serving size: *Vegetables:* 2 cups raw vegetables or 1 cup cooked. *Fruit:* 1 cup fresh fruit or ½ cup dried fruit or 1 medium sized fruit, like a medium apple

NUTS: Rich in vitamin E, an antioxidant that helps protect your brain, nuts are important for your cognitive health—and they make a great snack, topping, or addition to many dishes. In this book, we'll work with nuts including almonds, pecans, and walnuts. Enjoy a serving of nuts at least five times per week.

Servings: 5 servings a week, at least

Serving size: 1 ounce (see page 8 for serving size estimations)

BEANS: Not only are beans rich in protein and fiber, they are packed with B vitamins, which are essential for brain function and health. Beans are also low in fat and easy to incorporate into a variety of dishes. Here, we'll experiment with black beans, chickpeas, kidney beans, and more. Enjoy a serving of beans at least four times per week.

Servings: 4 servings per week, at least

Serving size: ½ cup cooked beans

WHOLE GRAINS: Essential fuel for your brain, the MIND Diet recommends three servings per day of whole grains. In this book, we'll explore recipes with oatmeal, quinoa, spelt, and many others.

Servings: 3 servings per day

Serving size: ½ cup cooked brown rice, whole grain pasta, steel cut oats, or other cooked grain; ½ cup cooked hot cereal, such as oatmeal; 1 slice 100 percent whole grain bread; 1 small whole grain muffin; 1 cup whole grain ready-to-eat cereal

SEAFOOD: Omega-3s are associated with a lower risk for Alzheimer's disease—and seafood is a great source of omega-3s. Some seafood are better sources: at least once per week enjoy a dish containing salmon, sardines, trout, or other seafood you enjoy.

Servings: 1 serving per week, at least

Serving size: 4 ounces cooked shrimp or other seafood, 6 ounces cooked fish

ADVICE ON EATING OUT

In today's world, there are an abundance of healthy, interesting options for when you want to go out to eat but still be in compliance with the MIND Diet. Avoid fast food restaurants (or ask for the salad option, with dressing on the side); rich, butter-laden foods; fried options; and most desserts (although most restaurants will have a fruit plate or sorbet option that you can enjoy). But you can still enjoy almost everything else. Think of the possibilities available to you that include whole grains, lean proteins, fresh vegetables, and luscious olive oil. After learning how to cook recipes from this book, you'll be comfortable finding options anywhere you go. We'll experiment with takes on what I call universal comfort food: dishes from home and a little bit from around the world. Think takes on Italian pastas, Thai curries, Southern stews, Southwestern tacos and burritos, and good old-fashioned favorites, like pizza, hummus, and coleslaw.

POULTRY: In addition to providing protein, an essential part of the diet, poultry contains vitamin B12, iron, and zinc, all of which are important for cognitive health

Servings: 2 servings per week (skin removed)

Serving size: 4 ounces

OLIVE OIL: Rich in over 230 anti-oxidant and anti-inflammatory properties, olive oil helps remove dangerous proteins from the brain. Since it has a lower smoke point, however, we use it either with low to medium low heat or as a finishing oil for salads and other cool dishes.

Servings: Use as your primary oil for low to low medium heat, or with cold dishes

Serving size: 1 tablespoon

WINE: A serving of wine (containing alcohol or not—either is fine) is recommended on the MIND Diet. Wine contains polyphenols, which are micronutrients that help prevent degenerative diseases.

Servings: 1 serving per day

Serving size: 5 ounces

Foods to Avoid

The five food groups to mainly avoid, or to indulge in sparingly, are the following:

RED MEATS: Consuming a lot of red meats such as beef, lamb, duck, and pork is associated with cognitive decline. Try to consume these less than four times per week, and when you do, look for lean, organic and/or grass-fed options, and the least processed cuts available. Processed foods like cured meats contain nitrites that can damage cells and also morph into molecules that cause cancer.

Servings: Less than 4, at most

Serving size: 3 ounces

PASTRIES AND SWEETS: As with most healthy diets, pastries and sweets should be enjoyed sparingly. On the MIND Diet, less than five times per week. Try to enjoy whole fruit, like berries, instead. When you have a sweet craving, however, enjoy the recipes in the Dessert section of this book. They were created as healthy alternatives to standard desserts.

Servings: 5 servings per week, at most

Serving size: 1 small cookie; 1 serving of other sweet, like ice cream

BUTTER AND STICK MARGARINE: Any fat that is solid at room temperature is a general no-no on the MIND Diet. Butter and stick margarine should be avoided, as well as palm oil, coconut oil, and shortening. Use olive oil or grapeseed oil as your fat. If you use butter, use it very sparingly.

Servings: Less than 1 per day

Serving size: 1 tablespoon

FULL-FAT CHEESE: Limit full-fat cheese to less than one serving per week. Better yet, opt for low- or no-fat options, which can be just as flavorful. Vegan cheese, which you'll find in the pages to follow, is a cholesterol-free option, and can be found at many grocery stores.

Servings: 1 serving per week, at most

Serving size: 1.5 ounces

FRIED OR FAST FOOD: Avoid fried and fast foods. The most you should have them is twice per month. Many restaurants, even fast food chains, have healthy options available, like salads or baked potatoes. It doesn't hurt to keep MIND-healthy snacks handy, like a baggie of nuts or a sandwich made on whole grain bread.

Servings: Twice a month at most

Serving size: 1 small serving of fries

Stocking the Pantry

In this book, you will find these common non-perishable ingredients and kitchen equipment. I've also included a few notes that may be helpful for your success on the MIND Diet. For a well-stocked kitchen, I recommend reading through the recipes and picking a few for the days or week ahead and shopping accordingly. These are some staples to get you started.

LOCAL HONEY: The bees in your area collect nectar from the plants that you're allergic to. By eating their honey, you can ingest tiny amounts of the allergens and build immunity to them.

NATURALLY SWEETENED OR LOW-SUGAR DRIED CRANBERRIES: You can find cranberries sweetened with apple juice at natural foods stores, or lower sugar versions at your local grocery store.

HERBS: Fresh or dried is fine, but dried lasts longer and tends to be more cost efficient. If you use fresh instead of dried, use about three times as much. Red pepper flakes, cinnamon, thyme, rosemary, basil, black pepper.

COOKING SPRAY: Find one that is not coconut oil and appropriate for the heat you will use. Remember, olive oil is best for low to medium, grapeseed for above.

WHOLE GRAINS: Steel cut oats, brown rice, whole grain pasta, quinoa

NUTS: Almonds, pecans, walnuts.

UNSWEETENED NON-DAIRY MILK: Soy, almond, cashew, or rice milk.

OIL: Extra-virgin olive oil for low to medium-low heat or finishing a dish. Grapeseed oil for cooking over medium and higher heat.

If possible, buy fresh ingredients. Frozen is next best, with canned being last. During the freezing process, food loses minimal nutritional value. When reheated, it becomes close to its "fresh" state again. When food is canned, however, we run into a few not-so-tasty factors: Nutrients may be damaged by the heating process, and the can's lining may contain Bisphenol-A, or BPA, a chemical that can migrate into your food and affect your health. Canned foods are also higher in sodium and preservatives. If you buy canned, make sure to drain the contents and then rinse them well.

COOKING TEMPERATURES

Chicken: Internal temperature should be at least 160°F to 165°F.

Fish: Internal temperature of fish should reach 145°F.

CHAPTER 1
BREAKFAST

You heard it from your mama first: Breakfast is the most important meal of the day. But you shouldn't have just any breakfast: A healthy breakfast, complete with protein, fiber, and vitamins and nutrients, can help jumpstart your productivity and your metabolism and nourish your brain. Breakfast foods are my favorite foods, and I've included some of my favorite recipes for you to enjoy here. Your brain uses the building blocks in your food to create the foundation for your day, and a good breakfast can help keep you focused throughout the morning and sharp until lunchtime.

Mind–Body Tip: Take a quick walk and enjoy the morning light. Your brain will wake up and adapt faster than it will sitting over a cup of coffee, and you can loosen up any stiffness from sleep.

OATMEAL "MUFFINS"

These "muffins" are what I grab when I'm in a rush but want something warm and comforting to eat. You can make a batch ahead of time and store them in the freezer. They will warm back into an oatmeal consistency upon being re-heated. Enjoy this tasty treat in a fraction of the time it takes to make regular, old-fashioned oatmeal, but with the same benefits. Try swapping out the blueberries for raisins or your favorite fresh or dried berries.

MIND foods: Whole grains, berries

Yield: 24 servings

Prep time: 5 minutes   **Cook time:** 30 minutes plus chill time

8 cups water	½ teaspoon cinnamon
¼ teaspoon sea salt	1 pint blueberries
2 cups steel cut oats	cooking spray
½ teaspoon local honey	

1. In a large pot, bring the water and salt to a rolling boil. Add oats, stir, and reduce heat to low. Cook for 30 minutes or until the water is absorbed and the oats are soft.

2. Turn off the heat and stir in the honey and cinnamon. Let the mixture rest for 10 minutes. Fold in the blueberries.

3. Use cooking spray to lightly grease two 12-cup muffin tins. Spoon in the oatmeal mixture.

4. Freeze flat for 5 hours or until solid.

5. Remove pans from the freezer. Using a butter knife or the edge of a spoon, gently pop the oatmeal "muffins" out of the tins. Place in a freezer bag, seal, and keep frozen for up to 3 months until ready to enjoy.

6. When ready to eat, place 1 or 2 "muffins" in a bowl and microwave for 2 to 3 minutes, stirring halfway through.

AVOCADO TOAST

Packed with healthy fats and spiced just right, this toast is light enough to not bog down your morning but hearty enough to help prepare you for the day ahead.

MIND foods: Whole grains, fruit, olive oil

Yield: 2 servings

Prep time: 5 minutes   **Cook time:** 3 minutes

4 slices whole-grain bread

1 ripe avocado

2 tablespoons olive oil

crushed red pepper flakes, to taste

salt and pepper

1. Toast the bread to desired crispiness.

2. Carefully cut the avocado in half, remove the seed, and slice the flesh into strips while still in skin.

3. Scoop out the avocado flesh with a spoon and divide the strips among the bread slices, spreading then lightly.

4. Drizzle the avocado toast lightly with the olive oil, then sprinkle with pepper flakes and salt and pepper, to taste.

AVOCADO TOAST WITH POACHED EGGS

Poached eggs add so much texture and protein to meals. Don't let them intimidate you—try it out! This dish is full of healthy fats and seasoned with a light sprinkle of basil.

MIND foods: Whole grains, fruits

Yield: 2 servings

Prep time: 5 minutes   **Cook time:** 5 minutes

4 eggs	salt and pepper, to taste
4 slices whole grain bread	¼ teaspoon basil
1 avocado, sliced	crushed red pepper flakes, to taste

1. Bring a medium pot of water to boil. Turn off the heat and carefully crack the eggs into 4 "corners" of the pot, not letting them touch. You can also use ramekins or oven-safe cups.

2. Cover the pot and poach for 4 to 5 minutes. Don't touch or stir the eggs. When done, gently remove with a slotted spoon. Set aside.

3. Toast the bread. Evenly divide the avocado slices between the slices of bread and gently spread the avocado slices like a butter.

4. Place the poached eggs on top of the toast. Sprinkle with salt, pepper, basil, and red pepper.

BLACK BEAN BREAKFAST BURRITOS

Who doesn't love burritos for every meal of the day? Warm and spicy, burritos for breakfast can be served with salsa, guacamole, hot sauce, or ketchup, or they are delicious on their own.

MIND foods: Beans, whole grains, vegetables, leafy green vegetables, olive oil

Yield: 6 servings

Prep time: 20 minutes   **Cook time:** 10 minutes

1 (15-ounce) can low-sodium black beans, rinsed and drained

¼ teaspoon ground cumin

¼ teaspoon chili powder

¼ teaspoon crushed red pepper flakes

1 tablespoon olive oil or cooking spray

10 eggs

6 whole wheat tortillas

3 small sweet potatoes, cooked and mashed

2 avocados, diced

1 cup chopped spinach

salt and pepper, to taste

1. In a large bowl, season the black beans with the cumin, chili powder, and crushed red pepper flakes. Set aside.

2. In a medium bowl, whisk the eggs together. Heat the olive oil or cooking spray in a large pan over medium-low heat. Add the eggs and cook for 3 to 4 minutes, stirring occasionally to scramble. Remove from heat and set aside.

3. Warm the tortillas in the microwave or the oven. Lay out the warm tortillas on a clean flat surface and evenly spread the mashed sweet potato on each. Next, evenly distribute the eggs, avocado, black beans, and spinach on each tortilla.

4. Season the burrito fillings with salt and pepper to taste. Tuck the ends of the tortillas in, then roll them up into burritos. Serve immediately.

VEGETABLE FRITTATA

A frittata sounds fancy, but it's surprisingly easy to make. Serve this dish to impress your family and friends at holiday events or for brunch. They'll never know how simple it was.

MIND food: Vegetables

Yield: 4 servings

Prep time: 10 minutes   **Cook time:** 20 minutes

8 eggs

¼ cup low-fat cheddar cheese, grated

½ cup halved cherry tomatoes

1 tablespoon chopped fresh basil

⅛ teaspoon black pepper

2 cloves garlic, minced

¼ teaspoon dried oregano

¼ teaspoon dried thyme

cooking spray

1 small yellow onion, thinly sliced

1 zucchini, chopped

10 asparagus spears, chopped into 2-inch pieces

1. Preheat the oven to 450°F.

2. In a large bowl, whisk the eggs well. Add the grated cheese, tomatoes, basil, pepper, garlic, oregano, and thyme, and set aside.

3. Heat a medium ovenproof, non-stick skillet to medium-high heat. Sauté the onion, zucchini, and asparagus for about 5 minutes or until the onion is translucent and the zucchini is browned. Remove from heat.

4. Pour the egg mixture into the skillet containing the vegetables, and stir once or twice to combine with vegetables. Place the skillet back over medium heat and cook for 2 more minutes, without stirring. Remove from heat.

5. Transfer the skillet to the oven. Cook for 12 to 15 minutes at 450°F or until a toothpick inserted into the center comes out clean.

PUMPKIN MUFFINS

I love pumpkin, and these muffins are so easy to make that I never have to wait until autumn rolls around to enjoy the taste. These are moist and yummy, and with the addition of chocolate chips, they can be a breakfast, sweet snack, or even dessert. Pumpkin also contains antioxidant vitamin C and potassium, which is vital for vascular health.

MIND foods: Vegetables, whole grains

Yield: 12 servings

Prep time: 10 minutes   **Cook time:** 25 minutes

cooking spray	1 teaspoon maple syrup
⅓ cup grapeseed oil	dash salt
½ cup local honey	½ teaspoon ground cinnamon
2 eggs	½ teaspoon ground ginger
1 cup unsweetened pumpkin puree	¼ teaspoon ground nutmeg
	¼ teaspoon ground allspice
¼ cup unsweetened nondairy milk	1¾ cups whole wheat flour
1 teaspoon baking soda	⅓ cup old-fashioned oats

1. Preheat the oven to 325°F. Grease a 12-cup muffin tin with cooking spray.

2. In a stand mixer or large bowl, beat the oil and honey together. Add the eggs and beat well.

3. Mix in the pumpkin puree and milk. Add the baking soda, maple syrup, and all of the spices, and combine.

4. Slowly add the flour and oats to the bowl and mix gently, until just combined.

5. Divide the batter evenly between the muffin cups. Bake for 20 to 25 minutes, or until the centers are firm.

6. Remove and let cool. Store covered, in the refrigerator, for up to 1 week.

LEMON BLUEBERRY MUFFINS

I made these once for a fancy brunch and, unfortunately for the host, who had spent hours cooking elaborate dishes, these muffins stole the show. They're tart and sweet and perfect to enjoy on your own—or to impress your friends.

MIND foods: Berries, whole grains

Yield: 12 servings

Prep time: 15 minutes   **Cook time:** 20 minutes

cooking spray	⅔ cup unsweetened nondairy milk
2¼ cup white whole wheat flour	1 teaspoon vanilla extract
2 teaspoons baking soda	⅔ cup local honey
1 teaspoon baking powder	½ cup grapeseed oil
pinch salt	1 cup blueberries, divided
1 lemon, juice and zest	

1. Grease a 12-cup muffin tin with cooking spray.

2. Preheat the oven to 350°F.

3. In a large bowl, whisk together the flour, baking soda, baking powder, and salt, and set aside.

4. In a medium bowl, whisk together the lemon zest and juice, milk, vanilla, and honey. Once combined, slowly whisk in the oil.

5. Add the wet mixture to the dry, and mix until combined. Don't overmix.

6. Gently fold in ⅔ cup blueberries.

7. Scoop the batter into the muffin pan. Top the muffins with the remaining ⅓ cup blueberries.

8. Bake for 18 to 20 minutes or until the centers are firm. (If you insert a toothpick into the middle and it comes out clean, the center is firm.)

QUINOA PORRIDGE

Porridge feels so old-fashioned and homey to me. Making it with quinoa, a complete protein, is a nice way to make this recipe modern, and it helps you feel full and satisfied.

MIND foods: Whole grains, berries, nuts

Yield: 4 servings

Prep time: 5 minutes   **Cook time:** 20 minutes

1 cup unsweetened nondairy milk

1 cup water

1 cup quinoa, rinsed

2 cups blueberries

½ teaspoon ground cinnamon

⅓ cup slivered almonds

4 teaspoons local honey

1. Combine the milk, water, and quinoa in a medium pot. Bring to a gentle boil over medium-high heat and then immediately reduce the heat to medium-low.

2. Cover and let simmer for 15 minutes, stirring occasionally, until most of the liquid is absorbed.

3. Remove the mixture from the heat and let stand, covered, for 5 minutes.

4. Stir in the blueberries and cinnamon. Serve topped with almonds and honey.

BANANA CHIP OVERNIGHT OATS

This is another great way to enjoy oats without waiting for them to cook in the morning. Sliced bananas and chocolate chips make this dish deliciously sweet, almost like banana muffins. The chia seeds and Greek yogurt pack a powerful protein punch.

MIND foods: Whole grains, berries

Yield: 2 servings

Prep time: 5 minutes plus chill time

⅓ cup low-fat Greek yogurt

½ cup steel cut oats

⅔ cup unsweetened nondairy milk

1 tablespoon chia seeds

½ teaspoon vanilla extract

dash of salt

2 tablespoons local honey

1 ripe banana, sliced

2 tablespoons dark chocolate chips

1. In a medium bowl, combine all the ingredients and gently stir. Pour into a medium mason jar, or 2 small mason jars, with a tightly fitting lid.

2. Refrigerate for 4 hours or overnight. Heat in the microwave or on the stove, or eat cold.

SAVORY OATMEAL WITH EGGS

This dish is so versatile, I've even eaten this oatmeal for dinner. Oats, eggs, mushrooms, and greens, this savory oatmeal is warming and hearty and wonderful for cozy mornings or nights.

MIND foods: Vegetables, whole grains, leafy green vegetables

Yield: 4 servings

Prep time: 5 minutes **Cook time:** 35 minutes

cooking spray

1 medium sweet yellow onion, chopped

8 ounces chopped baby bella mushrooms

1 clove garlic, minced

6 cups water

1½ cups steel cut oats

1 cup baby arugula

1 tablespoon grapeseed oil

4 eggs

1 avocado, sliced

salt and pepper, to taste

1. Spray a large skillet with cooking spray and heat over medium-high heat. Add the onion, mushrooms, and garlic, and cook for 6 to 7 minutes, stirring often. Remove from heat and set aside.

2. In a medium pot, bring the water to a boil. Add the oats, then immediately reduce heat to medium-low and simmer for 25 to 30 minutes. Stir in the arugula. Cover and let stand.

3. For fried eggs: While the oatmeal is cooking, heat the grapeseed oil in a medium skillet over medium-high heat. When the skillet is hot, crack the eggs onto the surface. Cook until the white is opaque and the yolk is the desired consistency.

3. For soft-boiled eggs: While the oatmeal is cooking, heat enough water to cover the eggs in a small pot over high heat. Bring the water to a boil, and then gently add the eggs. Boil for 7 minutes. Remove the eggs and either run them under cold water or place them in an ice bath to stop the cooking process. Peel gently.

4. Serve the oatmeal topped with the onion and mushroom mixture, avocado slices, and egg. Season with salt and pepper.

JOYFUL ALMOND OVERNIGHT OATS

We don't need to deprive ourselves to be healthy; we just need to find ways to make good choices. These overnight oats are truly joyful. The almond butter and chia seeds in this recipe help make this delicious breakfast a protein-packed treat.

MIND foods: Whole grains, berries, nuts

Yield: 2 servings

Prep time: 10 minutes   **Cook time:** 10 minutes plus chill time

1 cup steel cut oats

1 banana, sliced

1 tablespoon chia seeds

2 cups unsweetened nondairy milk

1 teaspoon vanilla extract

¼ cup almond butter

2 tablespoons dark chocolate chips

dash salt

1. Evenly divide the oats, banana, and chia seeds to two 10-ounce jars. Add the unsweetened nondairy milk and vanilla and gently stir.

2. Put the lids on and give the jars a good shake. Refrigerate for 4 hours or overnight.

3. When ready to eat, heat in the microwave or in a small pot on the stovetop, or eat cold.

4. To serve, top with the almond butter and dark chocolate chips and a dash of salt.

BREAKFAST TACOS

Tacos for breakfast can be a fun way to include family or children into cooking a meal. Create stations for your toppings and shells and let people create their own breakfast tacos for an interactive family meal.

MIND foods: Whole grains, beans, leafy green vegetables, vegetables

Yield: 4 servings

Prep time: 5 minutes   **Cook time:** 15 minutes

8 corn or whole wheat tortillas

cooking spray

4 eggs

½ cup cooked low-sodium black beans, rinsed and drained

¼ teaspoon crushed red pepper flakes

½ teaspoon garlic powder

1 cup spinach

1 avocado, sliced

1 cup Super Slaw (page 136) or red cabbage, shredded

1. Toast the tortillas on a medium heat grill or in the oven at 350°F until they reach desired warmth, for about 5 to 7 minutes.

2. Spray the bottom of a large skillet with cooking spray and heat over medium heat. Whisk the eggs in a small bowl and pour into the skillet. Lower the heat to medium-low and gently scramble.

3. Add the black beans and season with crushed red pepper flakes and garlic powder. Stir.

4. Add the spinach and stir, making sure to scrape the bottom of the skillet. Once the eggs begin to firm, remove from heat.

5. Place the egg mixture in the tortillas. Top with sliced avocado and either Super Slaw or shredded red cabbage.

SWEET POTATO FLORENTINE HASH

Hash is a great way to combine several ingredients into one flavorful dish. Throw in whatever veggies you have in your fridge to make hash a budget- and eco-friendly option. This colorful creation is full of fiber, brain-healthy vitamins (sweet potato is a great source of vitamin B6, which helps maintain the nervous system), and protein.

MIND foods: Vegetables, leafy green vegetables

Yield: 4 servings

Prep time: 5 minutes   **Cook time:** 10 minutes

2 tablespoons grapeseed oil

2 sweet potatoes, shredded

2 cups spinach, chopped

4 eggs

½ teaspoon crushed red pepper flakes

salt and pepper

1. Over medium-high heat, heat grapeseed oil in a large pan. Add shredded potatoes and cook for 5 minutes. Stir and cook for 2 minutes more, or until potatoes are cooked through.

2. Reduce heat to medium. Add spinach and stir, just until it begins to wilt.

3. Make 4 small wells in the sweet potato and spinach mixture. Crack 1 egg into each well.

4. Cover and reduce heat to medium-low. Cook for 2 to 3 minutes, or until eggs reach desired doneness. Season with red pepper, and salt and pepper to taste.

HOMEMADE BLUEBERRY MUESLI

Muesli can be very expensive to buy, and it tends to be eaten quickly in our house. No matter—it's more fun to make your own, anyway. With endless combinations, you can enjoy homemade muesli whenever you want. It's delicious plain, with low-fat Greek yogurt, or with unsweetened nondairy milk. Top with sliced bananas or fresh berries.

MIND foods: Whole grains, berries, nuts

Yield: 14 to 16 servings

Prep time: 5 minutes **Cook time:** 15 minutes

2 cups steel cut oats	¼ cup ground flax seeds
1 cup rolled spelt	3 tablespoons local honey
½ cup dried blueberries	1 teaspoon maple syrup
½ cup chopped almonds	½ teaspoon ground cinnamon
½ cup chopped pecans	

1. Preheat the oven to 350°F.

2. In a large bowl, combine the oats, spelt, blueberries, almonds, pecans, and flax seeds. Mix well.

3. Pour in the honey and maple syrup and toss to coat evenly. Sprinkle with cinnamon and toss well.

4. Pour the mixture evenly onto a baking sheet and bake for 15 minutes, stirring once halfway. Remove from heat and let cool.

WHOLE GRAIN BLUEBERRY PANCAKES

Sometimes, a day just calls for pancakes. You can still enjoy pancakes on the MIND Diet, and these are yummy, healthy, and have brain benefits from the oats and berries.

MIND foods: Whole grains, berries

Yield: 4 servings

Prep time: 10 minutes   **Cook time:** 20 minutes

2 cups whole wheat flour

1 cup quick/instant oats

dash salt

4 teaspoons baking powder

1 teaspoon ground cinnamon

4 egg whites

2 cups unsweetened nondairy milk

2 tablespoons local honey

½ cup low-fat Greek yogurt

1 teaspoon vanilla extract

1 cup blueberries with 1 tablespoon whole wheat flour

cooking spray

1. In a large bowl, combine the flour, oats, salt, baking powder, and cinnamon.

2. In a medium bowl, whisk the egg whites and unsweetened nondairy milk together. Add the honey and yogurt and whisk until no lumps remain. Add the vanilla and whisk until combined.

3. Make a well in the middle of the dry ingredients and slowly pour the wet ingredients in. Gently fold the wet ingredients into the dry. Mix until just combined; do not overmix.

4. If you're adding blueberries, coat them in 1 tablespoon of whole wheat flour to prevent them from bursting in your pancakes, and then gently fold them into the batter.

5. Coat the bottom of a large skillet with cooking spray. Heat it over medium.

6. Once the skillet is hot, use a ladle or large spoon to pour the batter, a bit at a time, onto the surface.

7. The bigger the pancakes, the more difficult they will be to flip. You will know it's time to flip when the edges of the pancakes look dry and bubbles start to appear in the middle. At this point, flip and cook on the other side for about 2 more minutes.

8. Remove the pancake from the heat and keep covered or in the oven to retain warmth.

9. Remove the pan from heat to carefully coat it with another layer of cooking spray. Return the skillet to the heat, then repeat steps 6 through 8 for the next pancakes.

10. Serve immediately.

HOMEMADE ALMOND JOY MUESLI

This homemade muesli mixture is full of flavor and provides a healthy start to the day. It also doubles as a nutritious snack. Serve plain, with low-fat Greek yogurt, or with unsweetened nondairy milk.

MIND foods: Whole grains, nuts

Yield: 6 to 8 servings

Prep time: 5 minute   **Cook time:** 15 minutes

4 cups steel cut oats	2 tablespoons maple syrup
1½ cups chopped almonds	1 tablespoon local honey
1½ cups unsweetened coconut flakes	1 tablespoon melted coconut oil
½ teaspoon ground cinnamon	½ cup chocolate chips

1. Preheat oven to 350°F.

2. In a large bowl, combine the oats, almonds, coconut, and cinnamon and mix well. Pour in the maple syrup, honey, and coconut oil, and mix well.

3. Pour the mixture evenly onto your baking sheet and bake for 15 minutes, stirring halfway.

4. Remove from heat and let cool. Let the muesli cool completely before mixing in the chocolate chips or you will make a muesli candy bar.

TOFU SCRAMBLE

This yummy Tofu Scramble is just as delicious as scrambled eggs—even if you've never considered tofu before. I make it all the time because it's that darn good. The spice turmeric, which gives it its bright yellow color, also has strong anti-inflammatory properties. You will be surprised at how egg-like it tastes, how easy it is to make, and how much you will enjoy it.

MIND food: Vegetables

Yield: 2 servings

Prep time: 5 minutes   **Cook time:** 10 minutes

1 block extra firm tofu

cooking spray

¼ teaspoon turmeric powder

½ teaspoon onion powder

½ teaspoon garlic powder

¼ cup low-sodium vegetable broth

salt and pepper, to taste

1. Drain the tofu and pat dry.

2. Spray a medium skillet with cooking spray and place over medium-high heat.

3. Season tofu with turmeric, onion powder, garlic powder, and salt and pepper. Add tofu to the skillet. Using a spoon or spatula, cut up the tofu in the pan to look like scrambled eggs.

4. As the tofu cooks, slowly add the vegetable broth to the mixture, letting it be absorbed into the mixture, stirring often.

5. The tofu will begin to brown. Once it does, remove from heat. Serve with whole grain toast.

HOMEMADE GRANOLA BARS

I have a granola bar at work every afternoon. It can be difficult, though, to find one that's not loaded with sugar and other not-so-great ingredients. I started making these as a way to get the quick, yummy snack I love without the ingredients I don't. As a bonus, they're cost effective and fun to make with kids.

MIND foods: Whole grains, nuts

Yield: 10 servings

Prep time: 20 minutes   **Cook time:** 15 minutes plus chill time

cooking spray

1½ cups steel cut oats

1 cup roasted unsalted almonds, chopped

¼ teaspoon cinnamon

1 packed cup medjool dates, pitted

¼ cup local honey

¼ cup Homemade Honey-Roasted Vanilla Bean Almond Butter (page 174)

¼ cup mini chocolate chips

1. Preheat the oven to 350°F. Spray a baking sheet with cooking spray.

2. Spread the oats and almonds on a baking sheet in a single layer. Season with cinnamon, and toast for 15 minutes. Remove and let cool.

3. In a food processor or high speed blender, blend the dates for about 1 minute, or until they form a doughy consistency.

4. In a large mixing bowl, combine the oats, almonds, and date mixture.

5. Over low heat, combine the honey and almond butter in a medium pot, stirring often. When it reaches a pourable consistency, after about 10 minutes, pour it over the oat mixture and mix it well.

6. Once mixed, transfer the mixture to a nonstick or greased baking dish. Press it into an even layer and let stand at room temperature.

7. Once the mixture is cool, sprinkle the chocolate chips over the top.

8. Cover the baking dish with plastic wrap and refrigerate for ½ hour, minimum.

9. Remove the mixture from the baking dish and chop into even squares. Store in an airtight container, refrigerated, for up to a week for a quick and easy breakfast.

ZUCCHINI BREAD

I remember the first time I realized the delicious bread I was eating was made from zucchinis. I was shocked and then delighted: vegetable bread? Zucchini Bread is so good, you'll doubt it's also good for you. But it is: zucchini contains zinc and niacin, which are essential for brain health. Dark chocolate contains flavonol, which helps reduce memory loss. Eat Zucchini Bread for breakfast, enjoy it as a snack, or bring it to a party—and it's up to you if you share the secret of how healthy your yummy bread really is.

MIND foods: Vegetables, whole grains

Yield: 12 servings

Prep time: 15 minutes   **Cook time:** 45 minutes to 1 hour

cooking spray (optional)

¾ cup unsweetened nondairy milk

2 eggs

¾ cup turbinado sugar

⅓ cup grapeseed oil

1 teaspoon maple syrup

2 small zucchinis, shredded

2 cups whole wheat flour

2 teaspoons baking powder

1 teaspoon cinnamon

dash salt

½ cup dark chocolate chips (optional) with 2 tablespoons whole wheat flour

1. Preheat the oven to 350°F.

2. Use a nonstick bread pan or spray a bread pan with cooking spray.

3. In a stand mixer or large mixing bowl, whisk together milk, eggs, sugar, oil, and maple syrup.

4. Stir in zucchini.

5. In a separate large bowl, combine flour, baking powder, cinnamon, and salt.

6. Slowly add the dry ingredients to the wet ingredients and stir until just combined.

7. If adding chocolate chips, fold in with whole wheat flour and gently fold into batter.

8. Pour the batter into the prepared pan. Bake for 45 minutes to 1 hour or until center is firm.

9. Remove and let cool.

GREEK YOGURT PARFAIT

Yogurt parfait is another easy option with endless flavor combinations. Make it with your favorite fruits (remember, berries are best for the MIND Diet!) and muesli or granola, and enjoy it for breakfast or a snack—or as a healthy dessert.

MIND foods: Whole grains, berries, nuts

Yield: 1 serving

Prep time: 5 minutes

1 cup plain low-fat Greek yogurt

1 cup Homemade Blueberry Muesli (page 29), or other muesli or granola

½ cup blueberries

½ banana, sliced

1. In a mason jar, small bowl, or large cup, layer ¼ cup of the yogurt on the bottom.

2. Top with ¼ cup of the muesli or granola, then 2 tablespoons each of the blueberries and bananas.

3. Repeat layering yogurt, muesli or granola, and fruits until ingredients run out.

NEW MEXICO BREAKFAST HASH

Years ago, I was driving through New Mexico and stopped to eat at a roadside diner, which was the only place I saw for miles that wasn't a gas station. I was so hungry, and the breakfast hash that I ordered was incredible. It also happened to be full of brain-healthy ingredients like bell peppers, sweet potatoes, and rosemary.

Mind food: Vegetables

Yield: 4 servings

Prep time: 10 minutes   **Cook time:** 20 to 22 minutes

2 tablespoons grapeseed oil

1 green bell pepper, seeded and chopped

1 medium yellow onion, chopped

4 sweet potatoes, chopped

1 tablespoon dried rosemary

4 eggs

salt and pepper, to taste

1. Preheat the oven to 400°F.

2. Coat a large cast iron or oven-safe skillet with the oil and heat over medium. Add bell pepper and onion and cook, stirring frequently, for approximately 5 minutes.

3. Season the potatoes with the rosemary, salt, and pepper, and add them to the skillet. Cook for 5 to 7 more minutes.

4. Remove the skillet from the heat. Make 4 wells in the hash mixture, leaving some hash at the bottom of the wells, and crack 1 egg into each.

5. Place the skillet in the oven and bake for 15 minutes. If you want a softer cooked egg, you can cook for less time, but check to make sure the potatoes are done.

VEGGIE OMELET

There are so many ways to add vegetables, and therefore nutrition, to your breakfast. Swap out the veggies suggested below for your favorite combinations whenever you want some variation.

MIND foods: Vegetables, leafy green vegetables

Yield: 2 servings

Prep time: 5 minutes   **Cook time:** 15 minutes

2 tablespoons grapeseed oil

½ red bell pepper, seeded and chopped

¼ medium sweet yellow onion, chopped

1 portobello mushroom, stem removed and chopped

1 clove garlic, minced

2 cups chopped spinach

4 eggs

¼ teaspoon crushed red pepper flakes

½ tablespoon dried basil

2 tablespoons water

salt and pepper, to taste

1. Heat 1 tablespoon grapeseed oil in a large pan over medium-high heat.

2. Add the bell pepper, onion, and mushrooms, and cook, stirring often, for 3 minutes, or until the onion is softened.

3. Add the garlic and stir to combine. Add the spinach and stir just until it wilts, about 30 seconds to 1 minute. Remove the mixture from the pan and set aside.

4. In a medium bowl, whisk together the eggs, red pepper, and basil.

5. For the first omelet, wipe out the pan and heat ½ tablespoon grapeseed oil over medium heat. Pour half of the eggs into the pan and let them thicken slightly over the bottom, approximately 2 to 3 minutes.

6. When the eggs begin to form a stiff surface, place half of the vegetable mixture over one half of the eggs.

7. Fold the other half of the eggs over the vegetables to make a pocket. Cook for 1 more minute. Remove from heat and set aside.

8. Repeat with the remaining eggs and vegetables. Season with salt and pepper. Serve with whole grain toast.

SCRAMBLED EGGS WITH SPINACH

The secret to great scrambled eggs is to cook the eggs very slowly over low heat for ultimate fluffiness. Add some spinach, for nutrients like folate and vitamin K, which have been shown to help with the brain's aging process and cognitive decline.

Mind food: Leafy green vegetables

Yield: 2 servings

Prep time: 5 minutes   **Cook time:** 5 minutes

cooking spray	¼ teaspoon garlic powder
4 eggs	3 cups chopped spinach
⅛ teaspoon crushed red pepper flakes	salt and pepper, to taste

1. Coat a medium skillet with cooking spray and heat over medium-low heat.

2. In a small bowl, whisk the eggs together. Season with red pepper and garlic powder. Pour into the skillet and keep heat medium-low to low. Stir occasionally, scraping the sides and bottom of the skillet.

3. Add the spinach when the eggs are still somewhat liquid, and fold them into mixture. Cook until the spinach is wilted and the eggs are set.

4. Remove from heat. Season with salt and pepper. Serve with whole grain toast.

HOLE IN ONE

This recipe combines two of my favorite foods in one awesome package. The trick with these is to scoop out a little more avocado than surrounds the pit and set it aside. Don't worry if the whites run over the edges—prop the avocados up in the baking dish and the eggs will still set. Use the leftover avocado as a yummy spread on your toast—the unsaturated fat in avocados help keep the cell membranes in your brain flexible.

Mind food: Fruit

Yield: 2 servings

Prep time: 5 minutes   **Cook time:** 15 minutes

1 avocado

2 eggs

salt and pepper, to taste

1. Preheat the oven to 450°F.

2. Cut the avocado in half and remove the pit. Scoop out a little bit of the avocado to make room for the egg, and set the removed flesh aside to add to the final dish.

3. Place avocado halves on a baking sheet with the hole facing up. Crack 1 egg each into the holes. Season with salt and pepper.

4. Bake for 10 to 15 minutes.

5. Serve with whole grain toast, using the scooped-out avocado as a spread.

CHAPTER 2
SMOOTHIES

Sometimes we can get so busy that we forget to consume all of the important nutrients we need for our brains and bodies. On those days, a smoothie comes in handy. But smoothies are so delicious, we don't need an excuse to enjoy them every day. Whatever your reason, a smoothie is a great way to get a lot of brain-healthy nutrients into one milkshake-like beverage. You can enjoy them on the go, or slowly sip and appreciate the flavors you've put together—and the brain benefits you're getting, too.

Note that my smoothies call for an optional cup of ice. 1 cup of ice will make a thicker smoothie but feel free to adjust this amount for your desired thickness.

Mind–Body Tip: Stretch. Gently reach for your knees or even your toes. Touch your elbow with your opposite hand. Give yourself a hug. Exercise, like stretching, may help regions of your brain that are key for memory retention and creating new cells. Stretch, and keep your body and brain limber.

BLUEBERRY BANANA SMOOTHIE

This smoothie is sweet and it's pretty, which is important as it makes you want to drink it! Enjoy this rich blend of antioxidants and omega-3s in a pretty purple smoothie. You can freeze bananas in advance for smoothies.

MIND foods: Berries, whole grains

Yield: 1 serving

Prep time: 5 minutes

1 banana, sliced

1 cup fresh or frozen blueberries

½ cup unsweetened nondairy milk or water

1 tablespoon chia seeds

1 cup spinach

1 cup ice (optional)

Add all ingredients to a blender and blend for 45 seconds or until liquefied.

SWEETHEART SMOOTHIE

Cherry season, one of my favorite times of year, was the inspiration for this blend. This smoothie is sweet and tart and has a wonderful, smooth mouth feel.

MIND foods: Leafy greens, berries, whole grains

Yield: 1 serving

Prep time: 5 minutes

½ avocado

1 cup kale

¼ cup fresh or frozen cherries

¼ cup fresh or frozen blueberries

1 banana

1 tablespoon chia seeds

1 cup unsweetened nondairy milk or water

1 cup ice (optional)

Add all ingredients to a blender and blend for 45 seconds or until liquefied.

BEACH SMOOTHIE

For a taste of the beach any time or anywhere on the MIND Diet, throw this smoothie in the blender. Tiny umbrella optional.

MIND foods: Berries, whole grains

Yield: 1 serving

Prep time: 5 minutes

1 cup unsweetened nondairy milk or water

1 banana

1 tablespoon ground flax seeds

1 tablespoon unsweetened coconut flakes

1 cup ice (optional)

Add all ingredients to a blender and blend for 45 seconds or until liquefied.

JUICE BOX SMOOTHIE

I loved juice boxes as a kid, but they're basically little sugar bombs devoid of nutrients. This smoothie delivers on the sweet taste while providing good fiber, as well as antioxidants and omega-3s.

MIND foods: Berries, whole grains

Yield: 1 serving

Prep time: 5 minutes

½ cup apple juice or water

1 banana

½ cup blueberries

1 cup raspberries

1 cup strawberries

1 tablespoon flax seeds

1 cup ice (optional)

Add all ingredients to a blender and blend for 45 seconds or until liquefied.

SWEET SPINACH SMOOTHIE

This spinach smoothie would make Popeye proud. The apple and apple juice makes it sweet and adds good fiber, while the spinach and avocado add healthy B vitamins and good fat.

Mind foods: Leafy greens, fruits

Yield: 1 serving

Prep time: 5 minutes

½ cup apple juice

½ cup water

1 cup spinach

½ apple, cored and chopped

¼ avocado

1 cup ice (optional)

Add all ingredients to a blender and blend for 45 seconds or until liquefied.

GREEN PINEAPPLE SMOOTHIE

Pineapple is one of my husband's favorite fruits, and I try to make things that include it whenever possible. This smoothie is loaded with whole-body benefits. Kale is high in iron, protein, and B vitamins, while pineapple is high in vitamin C and the bananas have potassium.

MIND foods: Leafy greens, berries

Yield: 1 serving

Prep time: 7 minutes

1 cup water

1 cup kale, stems removed and chopped

½ cup chopped pineapple

½ banana, chopped

1 cup ice (optional)

Add all ingredients to a blender and blend for 45 seconds or until liquefied.

SPICY SMOOTHIE

This spicy smoothie is spicy, but not overwhelmingly so, because I know most people aren't as spice-crazy as I am. The other ingredients keep it cool and even sweet, with little hints of spiciness throughout. Choose coconut water for a sweeter smoothie.

MIND foods: Leafy greens, vegetables

Yield: 1 serving

Prep time: 7 minutes

½ cup chopped spinach

½ mango, pitted and chopped

1 cup water or coconut water

½ cup chopped cucumber

⅛ to ¼ jalapeño, seeded and chopped

2 tablespoons fresh cilantro, chopped

1 sprig mint

½ lime, juiced

1 cup ice (optional)

Add all ingredients to a blender and blend for 45 seconds or until liquefied.

SWEET BEET SMOOTHIE

Remember our goal of pretty smoothies? You can't get much prettier than the gorgeous red of beets. Beets are full of phytonutrients and antioxidants, and may help reduce inflammation and lower your blood pressure. Enjoy this beautiful liver-detoxifier with ice or, as I prefer, at room temperature.

MIND foods: Berries, vegetables

Yield: 1 serving

Prep time: 10 minutes

1 cup unsweetened nondairy milk or water

½ banana, sliced

½ beet, washed, peeled, and chopped

½ cup chopped strawberries

½ cup blueberries

1 cup ice (optional)

Add all ingredients to a blender and blend for 45 seconds or until liquefied.

STRAWBERRY BANANA SMOOTHIE

This classic combination is packed with protein and healthy fat and tastes like a delicious (healthy) milkshake.

Mind foods: Berries, nuts

Yield: 1 serving

Prep time: 5 minutes

½ cup chopped strawberries

1 cup unsweetened nondairy milk or water

2 tablespoons almond butter

½ banana, sliced

1 cup ice (optional)

Add all ingredients to a blender and blend for 45 seconds or until liquefied.

DESSERT SMOOTHIE

This smoothie is so yummy that it tastes like dessert in a cup, which is where it gets its name. One of my favorite combinations, it's full of healthy fat, protein, and potassium. Local honey may help fight allergies and build up general immunity, plus it's a natural way to make things sweet.

Mind foods: Nuts, berries

Yield: 1 serving

Prep time: 5 minutes

2 tablespoons almond butter

1 cup unsweetened nondairy milk or water

½ banana, sliced

2 teaspoons local honey

1 cup ice (optional)

Add all ingredients to a blender and blend for 45 seconds or until liquefied.

CHAPTER 3

LUNCH

Ever notice that post-lunch slump where your blood sugar drops, productivity stalls, and you want to take a nap? I sure have, and it's not a great way to feel. Most likely, this happens when lunch consists of too many of the wrong kinds of foods. The right kinds of foods, like those found in the MIND Diet, will keep you alert, energetic, and feeling mentally sharp throughout the day. Pack your lunch with leafy greens, nuts, lean protein, and fiber. You won't experience that mid-afternoon slump, because who has time to lose a whole hour?

Mind–Body Tip: Another way to stave off that mid-afternoon slump is to go for a brisk walk. 120 minutes of exercise per week, which is less than 20 minutes per day, produces brain and body benefits.

WALNUT KALE SALAD WITH CHICKEN

Salad is a great way to enjoy a lot of flavors and textures in one delicious dish. This salad contains walnuts, which are a top nut for DHA, an omega-3 fatty acid that may help improve cognitive performance in adults, as well as prevent or slow down cognitive decline. This salad goes well with the Balsamic Dijon Dressing (page 160).

Mind foods: Poultry, nuts, leafy green vegetables, berries

Yield: 2 servings

Prep time: 20 minutes   **Cook time:** 25 minutes

2 boneless, skinless chicken breasts	¼ cup naturally sweetened or low-sugar dried cranberries
¼ cup raw walnuts	¼ cup crumbled goat cheese
8 cups loosely packed baby kale	½ medium ripe avocado, sliced
1 Bosc pear, chopped	salt and pepper, to taste

1. Preheat oven to 350°F.

2. Season chicken lightly with salt and pepper. Bake for 20 to 25 minutes or until cooked through. Set aside to cool. When cool, cut into bite sized pieces.

3. Chop walnuts into small pieces. Set aside.

4. In a large bowl, toss kale, pear, and cranberries together. Top salad with goat cheese, avocado, chicken, toasted walnuts, and dressing of your choice.

GRILLED CHICKEN PAILLARD

Chicken Paillard is another dish that only sounds fancy, but it is really quite simple. Paillard means "meat that has been pounded to be thin." So, if you have a meat mallet, or even a rolling pin, you can make this dish—and take out some frustration along the way.

Mind foods: Poultry, olive oil

Yield: 4 servings

Prep time: 10 minutes   **Cook time:** 10 minutes

4 boneless, skinless chicken breasts	½ teaspoon ground black pepper
2 tablespoons olive oil	¼ teaspoon garlic powder
½ teaspoon salt	½ teaspoon dried basil
	½ teaspoon dried parsley

1. Preheat the grill or a grill pan to medium-high.

2. Place each chicken breast between 2 sheets of wax paper or plastic wrap. Using a meat mallet or a similar utensil, pound the chicken evenly until it is approximately ¼-inch thick.

3. Brush both sides of each chicken breast lightly with olive oil.

4. In a small bowl, combine the salt, pepper, garlic powder, basil, and parsley, and sprinkle it evenly over both sides of the chicken breasts.

5. Grill the chicken, turning once halfway through (about 5 to 6 minutes on each side), until cooked through. Serve with a side of Strawberry Spinach Salad (page 71).

SPICY BLACK BEAN BURGERS

Vegetarian burgers can actually be quite flavorful and full of texture, without the added bad-for-your-brain fats that beef patties have. Enjoy this one on a whole-wheat bun or with greens.

MIND foods: Beans, vegetables

Yield: 4 servings

Prep time: 15 minutes   **Cook time:** 20 minutes

1 (16-ounce) can low-sodium black beans, rinsed and drained

½ red, green, or yellow bell pepper, minced

½ medium yellow onion, minced

3 cloves garlic, minced

1 egg

1 tablespoon chili powder

1 tablespoon ground cumin

1 teaspoon low-sodium Worcestershire sauce

½ cup bread crumbs

1. Preheat the oven to 375°F and grease a baking sheet.

2. In a large bowl, mash the black beans with a fork until they are thick and pasty. Add the bell pepper, onion, and garlic to the mashed beans.

3. In a small bowl, stir together the egg, chili powder, cumin, and Worcestershire sauce.

4. Stir the egg mixture into the mashed beans until combined. Mix in the bread crumbs until the mixture is sticky and holds together. Divide the mixture into 4 patties.

5. Place the patties on the baking sheet. Bake for 10 minutes and then flip. Bake for another 10 minutes, then remove from the oven and enjoy!

CREAMY TUNA SALAD

While the secret to this tuna salad recipe is the lemon juice, the brain-healthy benefits come from using a combination of low-fat Greek yogurt, avocado, and olive oil instead of mayonnaise. The probiotics in the yogurt may help protect your brain, while the monounsaturated fat in the avocado promotes blood flow to the brain and the olive oil helps protect against oxidative stress that can damage your cells and lead to cognitive decline.

MIND foods: Fish, vegetables, berries, nuts, olive oil

Yield: 2 servings

Prep time: 15 minutes

1 can albacore tuna (packed in water), drained

2 stalks celery, diced

1½ tablespoons naturally sweetened or reduced-sugar dried cranberries

1 tablespoon chopped toasted pecans

⅓ cup low-fat Greek yogurt

2 teaspoons olive oil

½ avocado, mashed

½ lemon, juiced

salt and pepper, to taste

1. In a medium bowl, combine the tuna, celery, dried cranberries, and pecans.

2. In a separate small bowl, stir together the Greek yogurt and olive oil. Add to the tuna and stir until combined.

3. Stir in the mashed avocado. Add the lemon juice and stir. Add salt and pepper to taste. Serve with crackers, on whole grain bread, or with salad.

WARM CHARD CHICKPEA SALAD

My sister has been making a version of this dish for several years as her go-to comfort food. It's quick and easy, and it can make a lot of people happy without a lot of fuss.

MIND foods: Vegetables, beans, leafy green vegetables, berries
Yield: 4 servings
Prep time: 5 minutes **Cook time:** 40 minutes

4 tablespoons grapeseed oil, divided

1 lemon, halved

1 medium sweet yellow onion, chopped

6 cloves garlic, minced

1 cup low or no-sodium chickpeas, rinsed and drained

1 cup water plus more, as needed

2 large bunches Swiss chard, ribs and stems removed, chopped

8 eggs

¼ teaspoon dried oregano

¼ teaspoon dried coriander

¼ teaspoon dried cumin

¼ teaspoon dried chili powder

¼ teaspoon crushed red pepper flakes

dash nutmeg

dash cinnamon

¼ cup naturally sweetened or reduced sugar cranberries

salt and pepper, to taste

1. Heat 2 tablespoons grapeseed oil in a medium pan over medium-high. Cut half of the lemon into slices and add them to the pan. Add half of the onion and a third of the minced garlic, and cook for about 4 minutes, stirring often. Zest and juice the remaining half of the lemon and set aside.

2. Add the chickpeas and the cup of water. Bring to a boil and stir.

3. Reduce heat, cover, and simmer for 5 minutes. Remove from heat and carefully discard most of the lemon and onion.

4. Over medium heat, heat 2 tablespoons of grapeseed oil in a large pan. Add the rest of the onion and garlic and cook for 5 minutes. Add Swiss chard and lemon zest and cook, stirring occasionally, for 5 to 8 minutes, or until chard is tender.

5. While the chard cooks, poach your eggs. Bring a large pot of water to boil. Turn off the heat and carefully crack the eggs into the "corners" of the pot (you can also use ramekins or oven-safe cups). Cover the pot and poach for 4 to 5 minutes. Don't touch or stir the eggs. When done, gently remove the eggs with a slotted spoon. Set aside.

6. Add chickpea mixture to the pan and stir. Add spices and stir to combine. Add more water if necessary. Add cranberries and stir well.

7. Reduce the heat to medium low. Let the mixture simmer for 3 to 5 more minutes, or until dish is combined.

8. Remove from heat. Serve topped with 2 poached eggs per serving. Sprinkle lemon juice to taste and season with salt and pepper.

COLORFUL THREE BEAN SALAD

The first time I made a bean salad, I didn't drain the beans. I was so confused by the murky, sticky concoction that I ended up with. Lesson: Drain and rinse your beans! Your bean salad will not only look better; it will taste better. And here's another tip: dry tomatoes with paper towels before chopping for a cleaner slice. Enjoy this salad for lunch or increase the recipe to bring to a picnic. This recipe pairs well with the Lemon Vinaigrette (page 177).

MIND foods: Beans, vegetables

Yield: 6 servings

Prep time: 15 minutes

1 (15-ounce) can low-sodium dark red kidney beans, drained and rinsed

1 (15-ounce) can low-sodium butter beans, drained and rinsed

1 (15-ounce) can low-sodium black beans, drained and rinsed

1 cup low-sodium canned, fresh, or frozen corn kernels

1 large tomato, seeded and chopped

1 small red onion, diced

½ green bell pepper, diced

½ cucumber, peeled, seeded, and diced

handful of fresh cilantro, chopped

Combine the beans, corn, tomato, onion, green pepper, cucumber, and cilantro in a large bowl and mix well.

SPICY CITRUS SHRIMP

I've always loved shrimp. Over the years, I've cooked it in so many different ways. Shrimp, like other seafood, has DHA, the omega-3 fatty acid that is good for your brain health. This recipe is low calorie and easy to make for a small group or for a large party. Serve with corn chips or salad for a full meal.

MIND foods: Vegetables, olive oil, fish

Yield: 4 servings

Prep time: 20 minutes

¼ cup chopped red onion

1 clove garlic, minced

2 limes, juiced

1 teaspoon olive oil

1 pound shrimp, cooked, peeled, and deveined

1 avocado, chopped

1 medium tomato, seeded and chopped

1 jalapeño, seeded and diced

handful fresh cilantro, chopped

salt and pepper, to taste

1. In a small bowl, combine the red onion, garlic, lime juice, olive oil, and salt and pepper. Let sit for at least 5 minutes.

2. Chop the shrimp and season with salt and pepper. In a large bowl, combine the shrimp, avocado, tomato, and jalapeño.

3. Combine all the ingredients together. If possible, cover and let it stand, refrigerated, for 30 minutes to an hour.

4. To serve, add cilantro and gently toss. Season with salt and pepper to taste.

NAWLINS RED BEANS AND RICE

A few years ago, my husband and I went to New Orleans for the beginning of Mardi Gras. I've never eaten so much delicious food. With a few adjustments, this New Orleans classic can be enjoyed without the unhealthy fats and salt. For a vegetarian twist, leave out the chicken sausage and substitute with vegetarian sausage or a soft-boiled egg.

MIND foods: Beans, poultry, vegetables, whole grains

Yield: 6 servings

Prep time: 1 hour   **Cook time:** 2 hours

1 pound dried red kidney beans

1 tablespoon grapeseed oil

½ pound andouille-style nitrate-free chicken sausage, thinly sliced

3 celery stalks, chopped

1 green bell pepper, chopped

1 medium sweet yellow onion, chopped

3 cloves garlic, minced

1 tablespoon Low-Sodium Blackening Seasoning (page 175)

1 bay leaf

8 cups water, plus more as needed

3 cups cooked brown rice, cooked according to package instructions

1. Place beans in a large pot and completely cover with water plus 2 inches more. Bring to a boil and cook for 1 minute.

2. Cover the beans and remove from heat. Let stand for 1 hour and then drain. Set aside.

3. When the beans have about 10 minutes or so left to soak, heat the grapeseed oil in a large pot over medium-high heat.

4. Add the chicken sausage, celery, bell pepper, and onion, and sauté 10 minutes, stirring frequently. Add the garlic and sauté 1 minute, stirring. Add the beans, blackening seasoning, bay leaf, and 8 cups of water.

5. Bring the mixture to a boil. Cover and reduce heat to low and simmer for 60 to 90 minutes, stirring occasionally, or until beans are tender.

6. Cook the rice according to package directions. Serve the red bean mixture over the rice.

KALE CAESAR SALAD

I love Caesar salads, and I wanted to find a way to make them healthier and more nutritious. So I thought, why not make something that tastes so good even better? The substitution of kale for romaine and the addition of chickpeas packs this salad with fiber, protein, iron, and B vitamins. Pistachios provide a great crunch and are a low-fat, low-calorie nut.

Mind foods: Whole grains, nuts, fish, olive oil, leafy green vegetables, beans

Yield: 2 servings

Prep time: 20 minutes

2 tablespoons grapeseed oil

4 cloves garlic, minced

¼ teaspoon crushed red pepper flakes

2 pieces of whole wheat bread, slightly stale if possible, cut into ½-inch cubes

¼ cup pistachios, shelled

½ cup grated Vegan Parmesan "Cheese" (page 170) or low-fat Parmesan

1 lemon, zest and juice

1 tablespoon Dijon mustard

1 teaspoon local honey

2 anchovy filets, cleaned and deboned

½ teaspoon Worcestershire sauce

¼ to ⅓ cup olive oil

salt and pepper, to taste

1 bunch of kale, stems removed and cut into strips

½ (15-ounce) can low or no-sodium chickpeas, drained, rinsed, and patted dry

1. Lightly coat a large sauté pan with grapeseed oil and heat over medium.

2. Add half the garlic, crushed red pepper, the bread cubes, and the pistachios. Cook, stirring often, until the bread and the garlic are golden brown and the pistachios are toasty, about 5 minutes.

Be careful not to burn the bread or nuts. Remove from the heat and set aside.

3. In a food processor or high speed blender, combine the cheese, lemon zest and juice, the remaining garlic, mustard, honey, anchovies, and Worcestershire sauce. Blend until the mixture is smooth, and while the machine running, add ¼ to ⅓ cup olive oil, until the dressing is the desired consistency. Season with salt and pepper as desired.

4. In a large bowl, toss the kale with the dressing, using your hands to massage the dressing into the kale. Let it rest for a minute. Add the croutons, chickpeas, and pistachios, and toss one last time to combine.

AVOCADO PESTO PASTA SALAD

Pesto is such a light and flavorful condiment. This avocado and walnut version is full of healthy fats and can be added to any pasta dish, or enjoyed with whole grain bread or crackers.

MIND foods: Nuts, olive oil, fruits, whole grains
Yield: 4 servings
Prep time: 15 minutes   **Cook time:** 20 minutes

½ avocado, sliced

¼ cup plus 1 tablespoon vegan or low-fat Parmesan

1 clove garlic, minced

1¼ cups fresh basil, divided

2 tablespoons raw walnuts

½ lemon, juiced

1 tablespoon olive oil

1 cup cherry tomatoes

½ bunch asparagus, sliced into 2-inch pieces, ends removed

½ medium zucchini, chopped

1 orange bell pepper, seeded and chopped

1 pound whole grain farfalle

salt and pepper, to taste

1. Combine the avocado, Parmesan, garlic, 1 cup basil, walnuts, lemon juice, and olive oil in a food processor or high speed blender and blend until smooth, about 30 seconds to 1 minute, depending on the food processor. Season with salt and pepper, to taste. Set aside.

2. Preheat the oven to 450°F.

3. Toss the vegetables in olive oil and season with salt and pepper, to taste. Roast for 20 minutes or until vegetables are tender.

4. Cook the pasta according to the package's instructions, about 10 minutes. Drain and rinse with cold water. Return the pasta to the pot.

5. When the pasta has cooled, toss with the avocado pesto. Top with roasted vegetables. Season with salt and pepper. Sprinkle basil to garnish.

PORTOBELLO SANDWICHES

Mushrooms are so meaty in texture, and they soak up any flavor you want to pair them with. Portobellos let you enjoy a meaty bite without the calories and weight of, well, meat. These are great for lunches or for picnics, with the bell peppers adding heat and sweetness, and the basil adding brightness.

MIND foods: Olive oil, vegetables, whole grains

Yield: 2 servings

Prep time: 10 minutes   **Cook time:** 10 minutes

2 tablespoons balsamic vinegar

1 tablespoon olive oil

1 clove garlic, minced

½ red bell pepper, seeded and sliced

2 portobello mushroom caps, stems removed

1 tablespoon grapeseed oil

¼ cup goat cheese, crumbled

4 slices whole grain bread, toasted

¼ cup chopped fresh basil

salt and pepper, to taste

1. Combine the balsamic vinegar, olive oil, and garlic in a large bowl. Add the bell peppers and portobello mushrooms and toss together until they are well coated in the mixture. Remove the vegetables from the mixture and set aside.

2. In a large skillet, heat grapeseed oil over medium heat.

3. Cook the bell peppers and mushrooms over medium heat for 4 minutes, stirring once, and then flip them over. Cook for 4 more minutes. Remove from heat.

4. Spread the goat cheese evenly onto 2 slices of toasted whole grain bread. Sprinkle with basil and season with salt and pepper.

5. Place 1 mushroom cap on top of each slice of cheese-coated bread. Top each cap with half of the bell peppers, then top with the second slice of bread. Press gently down and cut in half. Serve.

SLOW COOKER WHITE CHICKEN CHILI

When the weather is cold or rainy, there's nothing more homey than something bubbling away in the slow cooker. We often make a batch of this white chicken chili and leave it on overnight so that we can wake up to a house full of delicious smells and an easy-to-pack lunch.

MIND foods: Poultry, beans, vegetables

Yield: 8 servings

Prep time: 30 minutes   **Cook time:** 6 to 8 hours

2 pounds boneless, skinless chicken breasts

2 (15.5-ounce) cans of low-sodium great northern beans, drained and rinsed

2 cups of fresh, frozen, or low-sodium canned corn kernels, drained and rinsed

1 poblano pepper, seeded and chopped (for less heat, use a green bell pepper)

1 medium sweet yellow onion, chopped

4 cloves garlic, minced

1 teaspoon ground cumin

½ teaspoon onion powder

½ teaspoon garlic powder

1½ teaspoon chili powder

¼ teaspoon cayenne pepper

¼ teaspoon ground paprika

1 (14.5-ounce) can low-sodium chicken broth

1¾ cups water

1 lime, juiced

black pepper, to taste

1. Place chicken breasts, beans, corn, pepper, onion, garlic, and spices in the slow cooker.

2. Add the chicken broth and water, and then squeeze the juice of the lime over the mixture.

3. Cook on low for 6 to 8 hours. Try not to open the lid.

4. Before removing from slow cooker, shred the chicken using forks. Stir the mixture thoroughly.

STRAWBERRY SPINACH SALAD

A strawberry spinach salad is one of my favorite things to order when I'm out to eat. Make this adapted MIND Diet version at home and bring it with you to work or wherever you would like to enjoy it.

MIND foods: Leafy green vegetables, berries, nuts, olive oil

Yield: 4 servings

Prep time: 10 minutes   **Cook time:** 3 minutes

3 cups baby spinach	¼ cup goat cheese, crumbled
3 cups arugula	½ avocado, diced
½ cup chopped pecans	2 tablespoons olive oil
2½ cups sliced fresh strawberries	½ lemon, juiced
	salt and pepper, to taste

1. Toss spinach and arugula together to combine.

2. Toast pecans in a small skillet over medium-low heat for 2 to 3 minutes, or until slightly browned. Be careful not to burn them. Remove from heat and set aside.

3. Top greens mixture with strawberries, toasted pecans, goat cheese, and avocado. Drizzle with olive oil and lemon juice. Season with salt and pepper. Toss to combine.

WARM FARRO SALAD

This recipe is another one that my sister, a long-time vegetarian, counts on when she wants to please a lot of people in a short amount of time. This warm salad is layered with so many flavors and textures, from hearty mushrooms to tart dried cranberries, you and the people you share this with are sure to discover flavors that you love.

MIND foods: Whole grains, olive oil, vegetables, leafy green vegetables, berries

Yield: 4 servings

Prep time: 20 minutes   **Cook time:** 35 minutes

2 cups uncooked farro

water, as needed

3 tablespoons plus 1 teaspoon olive oil, divided

1 tablespoon balsamic vinegar

1 tablespoon apple cider vinegar

1 tablespoon local honey

1 tablespoon grapeseed oil

1 pound baby bella mushrooms

1 bunch dinosaur kale, stems removed and chopped

2 teaspoons dried thyme

¼ cup naturally sweetened or reduced-sugar dried cranberries

6 tablespoons goat cheese, crumbled

2 tablespoons dried parsley

salt and pepper, to taste

1. Cook farro according to package instructions, about 30 minutes in boiling water. You can soak your farro overnight beforehand if you'd like, but it's not necessary. Drain, toss with 1 teaspoon of olive oil to keep from sticking, and set aside.

2. In a small bowl, whisk together the balsamic vinegar, apple cider vinegar, honey, and 3 tablespoons olive oil. Set aside.

3. Heat 1 tablespoon grapeseed oil over medium-high heat and add the mushrooms. Cook for 3 to 4 minutes, stirring occasionally. Add the kale and season with thyme.

4. Cook for 1 to 2 minutes more, or until kale is softened. Remove from heat.

5. In a large bowl, combine the farro, cranberries, mushrooms, and kale. Sprinkle with goat cheese and parsley, and drizzle with the dressing you made to taste. Season with salt and pepper.

TUNA WRAP

My grandma's Creamy Tuna Salad (page 59) is one of my favorite lunches, but it can be messy. A wrap is a great way to enjoy it without making a mess. Enjoy healthy fats, protein, and antioxidants in this dish.

MIND foods: Whole grains, fish, leafy greens, vegetables

Yield: 4 servings

Prep time: 5 minutes

4 whole wheat wraps	1 avocado, sliced
1 recipe Creamy Tuna Salad (page 59)	1 carrot, sliced into matchsticks
2 cups chopped spinach	salt and pepper, to taste

1. Spread the wraps on a clean flat surface.

2. Spread ¼ of the Creamy Tuna Salad over each wrap. Season with salt and pepper.

3. Top with spinach, avocado slices, and carrot strips. Roll up the wraps and cut them in half to serve.

T-BLAT

A BLT has to be one of the most satisfying and delicious sand-wiches I've ever tasted, but it's full of nitrates and unhealthy fat. The T-BLAT, however, is full of good protein, healthy fat, and even antioxidants and fiber. Satisfying, delicious, and healthy. Toast the bread for an added crunch.

MIND foods: Poultry, vegetables, whole grains, leafy green vegetables

Yield: 4 servings

Prep time: 15 minutes   **Cook time:** 10 minutes

8 slices all-natural, nitrate-free turkey bacon

1 avocado

2 tablespoons dried basil

½ teaspoon garlic powder

¼ teaspoon crushed red pepper flakes

8 slices whole grain bread

1 medium tomato (heirloom if in season), sliced

4 leaves romaine, trimmed to size

salt and pepper, to taste

1. In a large skillet, cook the turkey bacon over medium heat for 7 to 10 minutes, or until crispy.

2. Remove the turkey bacon from the heat and drain oil. Pat dry with paper towels.

3. In a medium bowl, mash the avocado with a fork. Season with the basil, garlic powder, and red pepper.

4. Spread the avocado mixture evenly on four slices of bread. Top evenly with bacon, tomato slices, and romaine lettuce. Season with salt and pepper. Top with the remaining pieces of bread.

SOUTHWEST SALAD

I like to make this salad and keep all of the ingredients separate in the bowl so that I can enjoy the beautiful colors before mixing them up together. There is so much flavor and texture going on in this salad, it's like several meals in one. Jicama, which may be an unfamiliar ingredient, is a mild root vegetable with benefits including fiber, vitamin C, E, several B vitamins, folate, and minerals like potassium, magnesium, manganese, copper, iron, and a small amount of protein.

MIND foods: Leafy green vegetables, beans, vegetables

Yield: 4 servings

Prep time: 10 minutes

6 cups spinach

2 cups arugula

2 cups kale, chopped or torn

2 (8-ounce) cans low-sodium black beans, rinsed and drained

1 (8-ounce) can low-sodium corn, rinsed and drained

2 cups grape tomatoes, halved

1 jicama, peeled and diced

1 recipe Southwest Dressing (page 158)

salt and pepper, to taste

1. Combine greens in a large bowl and mix well.

2. Divide the greens into 4 serving bowls or plates. Top greens with the black beans, corn, tomatoes, and jicama. Season with salt and pepper. Serve with 1 cup Southwest Dressing.

CORNIGLIA SARDINES

Sardines are often an unappreciated brain booster. Charged with EPA and DHA, omega-3 fatty acids, sardines can help your brain cells communicate better, keeping the neurotransmitters responsible for mental focus in prime condition.

MIND foods: Olive oil, fish

Yield: 2 to 4 servings

Prep time: 30 minutes to 1 hour   **Cook time:** 10 minutes

4 medium cloves garlic, finely minced

¼ cup olive oil

2 lemons, 1 juiced and 1 cut into wedges

1 teaspoon smoked paprika

1 pound fresh sardines, cleaned, scaled, and gutted

2 tablespoons dried parsley

salt and pepper, to taste

1. Combine the garlic, olive oil, lemon juice, paprika, and pepper in a small bowl and whisk to combine.

2. Spread the sardines in a single layer on the bottom of a baking dish and pour the mixture over the fish, ensuring they are coated evenly. Marinate for 30 minutes to 1 hour.

3. Preheat a gas grill to high heat, or preheat the oven to 450°F.

4. If grilling the sardines, grill them over direct heat for 2 to 3 minutes on each side. If baking, bake for 8 to 10 minutes.

5. Serve sprinkled with parsley and with lemon wedges on the side. Season with salt and pepper as desired.

RAINY DAY MINESTRONE

Minestrone soup is a nice cold weather dish. I love whole wheat, low-sodium crackers to pair with it. It doesn't take long to make, and it takes the chill out as I wait for the warmer weather to arrive.

MIND foods: Vegetables, whole grains, leafy green vegetables, beans

Yield: 4 to 6 servings

Prep time: 10 minutes   **Cook time:** 1 hour

cooking spray

3 cloves garlic, minced

1 small white onion, diced

2 medium-large carrots, peeled and sliced

2 pounds tomatoes, peeled, seeded, and diced

4 cups water

¼ cup uncooked quinoa

½ teaspoon dried basil

½ teaspoon dried rosemary

½ teaspoon dried parsley

dash marjoram

2 bay leaves

black pepper, to taste

1 small zucchini, chopped

½ bunch (approximately 10) spears asparagus, chopped into 1-inch pieces

1 packed cup chopped kale or spinach

1 (15-ounce) can low or no-sodium white beans, rinsed and drained

½ cup peas, frozen

vegan or low-fat cheese, to garnish

1. Coat the bottom of a large sauce pot with cooking spray and heat over medium-high heat.

2. Add garlic, onion, and carrot, and sauté until they start to brown.

3. Add tomatoes, water, quinoa, spices, bay leaves, and pepper, and stir to combine.

4. Bring the mixture to a boil and cover. Reduce to a simmer and cook for 30 minutes.

5. Add the remaining vegetables and beans. Cook for 20 minutes more until asparagus has started to soften, but is still vibrantly green.

6. Remove from heat and serve, garnishing with vegan or low-fat cheese.

FANCY BALSAMIC PRIMAVERA

Chock full of delicious, colorful vegetables, giving you fiber, antioxidants, and vitamins galore, this is an inexpensive and easy-to-make dish. Serve warm or chilled.

MIND foods: Vegetables, olive oil, whole grains
Yield: 4 servings
Prep time: 15 minutes   **Cook time:** 30 minutes

2 cups chopped broccoli

1 cup halved cherry or grape tomatoes

1 cup chopped portobello mushrooms

1 orange or yellow bell pepper, cored and chopped

5 tablespoons olive oil, divided

1 teaspoon dried basil

16 ounces whole grain bow tie pasta

cooking spray

3 cloves garlic, minced

¼ cup balsamic vinegar

handful of fresh basil leaves

¾ cup grated Vegan Parmesan "Cheese" (page 170), low-fat grated cheese, or nutritional yeast

salt and pepper, to taste

1. Preheat the oven to 450°F. In a large bowl, toss the broccoli, tomato, mushroom, and bell pepper with 3 tablespoons of olive oil and season with dried basil, salt, and pepper. Bake for 15 to 20 minutes.

2. Cook the pasta according to package instructions until it's al dente, about 8 minutes. Drain the pasta and reserve 1 cup of pasta water.

3. Coat a large pan with cooking spray. Cook the garlic over medium-high heat until browned. Add the drained pasta. Add a little bit of pasta water. Stir gently to combine. Add the roasted vegetables and stir.

4. Cook for 3 minutes, stirring occasionally, over medium heat, adding pasta water as needed to thin the mixture.

5. Turn the heat to medium-high, cook for 1 more minute, and then pour the balsamic vinegar over the mixture. Give it one final stir and remove from heat.

6. Serve with fresh basil and vegan Parmesan, nutritional yeast, or low-fat cheese.

EASY VEGGIE WRAP

This is a great light option, another recipe from my time as a vegan. Seasoned with an Italian flair, this wrap is full of fiber and healthy veggies.

MIND foods: Vegetables, olive oil, whole grains, leafy green vegetables

Yield: 4 servings

Prep time: 20 minutes

1 (14-ounce) can low-sodium artichoke hearts, rinsed, drained, and chopped

1 tomato, seeded and diced

2 tablespoons balsamic vinegar

1 tablespoon olive oil

½ teaspoon crushed red pepper flakes

½ teaspoon dried basil

1 teaspoon dried oregano

4 whole grain wraps

½ small red onion, thinly sliced

2 cups spinach

salt and pepper, to taste

1. In a medium bowl, combine the artichoke hearts, tomato, vinegar, oil, red pepper, basil, and oregano. Toss to coat evenly.

2. Spread the wraps on a clean flat surface and evenly divide the vegetable mixture between them. Top with the onion and spinach. Season with salt and pepper.

3. Fold the bottoms up. Roll the wraps over the mixture firmly to enclose the fillings. They should be wrapped tightly enough to not unroll, but if not, spear in the middle with a toothpick.

SALMON TACOS

Salmon tacos scream "summer" to me. Fortunately, you don't need to wait until summer to enjoy this satisfying, flavorful dish. Try it with Mango Guacamole (page 176) or Roasted Garlic Guacamole (page 159) and see which one you like better.

MIND foods: Fish, vegetables

Yield: 4 servings

Prep time: 10 minutes   **Cook time:** 20 minutes

1 tablespoon Low-Sodium Blackening Seasoning (page 175)

1 pound fresh salmon filets

cooking spray

1 cup shredded red cabbage

8 corn or whole grain tortillas

1. Preheat oven to 400°F.

2. Sprinkle the Low-Sodium Blackening Seasoning on the non-skin side of the salmon, making sure to coat evenly. Spray a large baking sheet with cooking spray and place the salmon skin-side down.

3. Bake for 15 to 20 minutes or until salmon is medium well and medium-light pink in color.

4. Remove from the oven and let cool. Flake the salmon with a fork and discard the skin.

5. Add the salmon and cabbage to tortillas. Serve with Mango or Roasted Garlic Guacamole.

SLOW COOKER JAMBALAYA

This version of the New Orleans favorite is lower in sodium, full of protein and veggies but still packed with flavor and spice, so you can enjoy it and not feel full and heavy after eating. Serve with fiber-full brown rice.

MIND foods: Poultry, vegetables, whole grains, fish

Yield: 8 servings

Prep time: 15 minutes   **Cook time:** 6 to 8 hours

1 pound boneless, skinless chicken breasts, cut into bite sized pieces

1 medium sweet yellow onion, chopped

1 green bell pepper, seeded and chopped

4 stalks celery, chopped

4 cups water

1 tablespoon dried oregano

1 tablespoon Low-Sodium Blackening Seasoning (page 175)

1 teaspoon crushed red pepper flakes

1 teaspoon dried thyme

1 bay leaf

2 (15-ounce) cans low-sodium diced tomatoes

2 cups cooked brown rice, cooked according to package instructions

1 pound raw shrimp, peeled, deveined, tails removed

1 tablespoon fresh parsley, chpped

salt and pepper, to taste

1. Set the slow cooker to low. Combine all ingredients in the slow cooker, except the brown rice, shrimp, and parsley, and cook for 6 to 8 hours.

2. Right before you're ready to eat, add the shrimp to the slow cooker. Cover and cook for 15 to 20 minutes or until the shrimp is cooked through. The shrimp should be opaque and pinkish white—if translucent, it means the shrimp is still raw; if too white, it's overcooked.

3. Mix with cooked brown rice before serving. Sprinkle with parsley.

CHAPTER 4

DINNER

Dinner is often our last opportunity to eat until breakfast. It's important to eat a well-balanced dinner so that our brains and our bodies have enough fuel to last until that next meal; otherwise, we risk blood sugar crashes and waking up in the middle of the night. Dinner is also a chance to spend time with our loved ones—or with ourselves. There are few things I love more than cooking a favorite meal and then sharing it with my family, or enjoying it quietly with a good book.

Mind–Body Tip: Make sure your bedroom is primed for a good night's sleep: no screens, bright lights, or noise. Try to sleep for at least seven hours to give your body and brain time to restore.

GARLICKY SHRIMP

This rich and flavorful dish pairs well with a whole grain like couscous, millet, or brown rice. You may not have tried halloumi before, but you can usually find it in your local grocery store. This semi-hard, unripened brined cheese from Cyprus is made from a mixture of goat's and sheep's milk, and can be grilled easily due to its high melting point. Try this dish with the Lemon Couscous (page 134).

MIND foods: Vegetables, fish, leafy green vegetables

Yield: 4 to 6 servings

Prep time: 20 minutes   **Cook time:** 15 minutes

1 pound raw shrimp, peeled, deveined, tails removed

¼ teaspoon crushed red pepper flakes

⅛ teaspoon chili powder

2 tablespoons grapeseed oil

½ shallot, chopped

3 cloves garlic, minced

1 red bell pepper, seeded and chopped

½ block halloumi cheese, sliced into cubes

1 bunch fresh spinach, chopped

½ lemon, juiced

¼ cup parsley, chopped

1. Pat shrimp dry. In a medium bowl, season the shrimp with red pepper and chili. Set aside.

2. Heat 1 tablespoon of grapeseed oil in a large pan over medium-high heat. Add the shallot and cook for 2 minutes, stirring often. Add the garlic and cook for 1 more minute, stirring often. Remove from heat and set aside in a small bowl.

3. Wipe out the pan. Heat 1 tablespoon of grapeseed oil over medium-high heat. Add the red pepper and halloumi. Cook for 5 to 7 minutes, stirring occasionally, or until halloumi is browned on both sides.

4. Turn the heat down to medium. Add the shrimp and stir. Add the shallot and garlic mixture and stir. Cook for 2 minutes.

5. Add the spinach and stir to combine. Cook for 1 minute, or until the spinach is barely wilted. Remove from heat.

6. Sprinkle with lemon juice and parsley to serve.

DIJON CHICKEN

Dijon mustard is tangy and sweet, all in one bite. Enjoy this flavorful, protein-packed dish with your favorite side like Honey-Glazed Carrots (page 146).

MIND food: Poultry

Yield: 4 servings

Prep time: 10 minutes   **Cook time:** 20 minutes

3 cloves garlic, minced

½ cup whole grain Dijon mustard

½ teaspoon paprika

2 tablespoons chopped fresh tarragon

4 boneless, skinless chicken breasts

salt and pepper, to taste

½ lemon, juiced

1. Preheat the oven to 425°F.

2. In a small bowl, whisk together the garlic, mustard, paprika, and tarragon. Set aside.

3. Season the chicken with salt and pepper on both sides.

4. Coat the chicken with the mustard mixture. Bake for 20 minutes or until cooked through. You can use a meat thermometer to check for doneness (internal temperature should be 160°F to 165°F) or cut a piece in half and check to ensure that the inside is white, not pink. Sprinkle with lemon juice before serving.

CREOLE SHRIMP

Another Southern favorite, this spicy shrimp dish delivers on flavor without packing a high-sodium punch. Serve with brown rice.

Mind foods: Vegetables, fish

Yield: 4 servings

Prep time: 15 minutes   **Cook time:** 35 minutes

2 tablespoons grapeseed oil

⅔ cup chopped sweet yellow onion

⅔ cup chopped celery

⅔ cup chopped green pepper

2 cloves garlic, minced

2 (15-ounce) cans low-sodium diced tomatoes, drained

1 cup water

2 (8-ounce) cans low-sodium tomato sauce

2 tablespoons low-sodium Worcestershire sauce

2 teaspoons local honey

dash salt

1 teaspoon chili powder

1 teaspoon ground paprika

1 pound raw shrimp, peeled, deveined, tails off

¼ cup chopped fresh parsley

1. In a large skillet, heat the grapeseed oil over medium and sauté the onion, celery, and green pepper until softened, about 5 minutes. Add garlic and sauté 1 minute longer.

2. Stir in the tomatoes, water, tomato sauce, Worcestershire sauce, honey, salt, chili powder, and paprika. Bring to a boil.

3. Reduce heat to medium low and simmer, uncovered, for 20 to 25 minutes, stirring occasionally.

4. Add the shrimp and cook for 5 minutes longer, or until the shrimp turns opaque and pinkish white—if translucent, it means the shrimp is still raw; if too white, it's overcooked.

5. Serve, sprinkled with parsley.

CRISPY SZECHUAN TOFU

A lot of people are afraid of trying tofu either because they've never made or tasted it before, or because they assume it's going to be soft or mushy. When I was vegan, I learned how to make tofu both crispy and delicious. Also, one of the good things about tofu is that it will take on almost any flavor you want.

MIND food: Vegetables

Yield: 4 servings

Prep time: 10 minutes   **Cook time:** 10 minutes plus chill time

1 pound extra firm tofu	½ teaspoon ginger
3 tablespoons low-sodium soy sauce	¼ teaspoon crushed red pepper flakes
2 tablespoons toasted sesame oil	2 tablespoons grapeseed oil
2 tablespoons apple cider vinegar	1 recipe Szechuan Vegetables (page 142)
1 teaspoon garlic powder	salt and pepper, to taste

1. Drain the tofu and pat dry. Season with salt and pepper.

2. Using a sharp knife, gently press down on the top of the tofu and carefully slice horizontally so that you have 2 thinner blocks. Next, slice the tofu into bite-sized cubes.

3. Place the tofu in an airtight container and freeze for at least an hour. The longer you freeze it, the crispier it will be when you cook it.

4. Remove from the freezer once you're ready to cook.

5. Combine all the remaining ingredients except for the grapeseed oil, salt and pepper, and Szechuan Vegetables in a small bowl and whisk to combine. Pour over the tofu, but leave a little bit to the side.

6. Heat the grapeseed oil in a large skillet over medium-high heat. Add the tofu and use a wooden or flat spatula to gently break the cubes apart. Cook, stirring occasionally. Add the liquid you retained after about 5 minutes, pouring it over the mixture and stirring to combine. Cook until the tofu is crispy and browned on all sides, for another 10 minutes.

7. Add Szechuan Vegetables to the skillet and heat for an additional two minutes to mix flavors.

WALNUT-CRUSTED CHICKEN

The walnuts in this recipe are a great way to get omega-3s, plus they provide a wonderful crunch to this well-seasoned chicken dish. Serve with Citrus Garlic Green Beans (page 145).

Mind foods: Poultry, olive oil, nuts, whole grains

Yield: 4 servings

Prep time: 4½ hours   **Cook time:** 25 minutes

4 chicken breasts, boneless and skinless

⅓ cup olive oil

¼ cup plus 3 tablespoons whole grain Dijon mustard, divided

¼ cup white wine

4 cloves garlic, minced

1 teaspoon dried thyme

2 cups raw walnuts, chopped

1 cup whole wheat flour

salt and pepper, to taste

2 tablespoons grapeseed oil

2 tablespoons dried parsley

⅓ cup local honey

1. Combine the chicken, olive oil, ¼ cup mustard, white wine, garlic, and thyme in an air-tight container or sealed bag. Refrigerate for 4 hours or overnight.

2. When you're ready to cook, preheat the oven to 425°F.

3. Combine the walnuts, flour, salt, and pepper together in a shallow baking dish. Dip the chicken into the walnut mixture and coat it evenly. Set aside.

4. Heat 2 tablespoons of grapeseed oil in a large oven-safe skillet over medium-high heat. Add the chicken and cook for 2 minutes on each side.

5. Transfer the skillet to the oven and bake for 20 minutes, or until the chicken is cooked through. You can use a meat thermometer to check for doneness (internal temperature should be 160°F to 165°F) or cut a piece in half and check to ensure that the inside is white, not pink.

6. Remove from the oven and let cool.

7. In a small bowl, whisk together the honey and 3 tablespoons mustard. Drizzle over the chicken, sprinkle with parsley, and serve.

SPICED CHICKEN

Spices not only make a dish more flavorful, but many spices also have brain health benefits. A flavonoid in some spices, like thyme, contains brain-boosting power that may help strengthen connections between neurons. Thyme has also been shown to increase the amount of DHA, an omega-3 fatty acid, in the brain. Garlic, along with warding off any pesky vampires, may help promote better blood flow to the brain.

Mind food: Poultry

Yield: 4 servings

Prep time: 10 minutes   **Cook time:** 10 minutes

2 teaspoons ground paprika	¼ cup balsamic vinegar
1 teaspoon ground cumin	2 tablespoons local honey
1 teaspoon dried thyme	4 boneless, skinless chicken breasts
1 clove garlic, minced	
	salt and pepper, to taste

1. Preheat the oven to 425°F.

2. In a small bowl, combine the paprika, cumin, thyme, and garlic. In another small bowl, whisk together the vinegar and honey.

3. Season the chicken with salt and pepper on both sides. Place the chicken in a baking dish, and pour the honey mixture over the chicken to coat. Then coat the chicken with the seasoning mixture on both sides.

4. Bake for 20 minutes, or until cooked through. You can use a meat thermometer to check for doneness (internal temperature should be 160°F to 165°F) or cut a piece in half and check to ensure that the inside is white, not pink.

GRANDMA'S MAC 'N' CHEESE

Macaroni and cheese is another dish that can be made healthier, and MIND-diet–friendlier, with a few simple tweaks. Use whole grain pasta and add fresh spinach for a little more nutrition and fiber. Replace the milk with low-fat Greek yogurt, and use low-fat cheese. Choose a pasta like elbows, penne, rigatoni, or rotini for this recipe.

Mind foods: Whole grains, leafy green vegetables

Yield: 6 to 8 servings

Prep time: 10 minutes   **Cook time:** 20 minutes

1 pound whole wheat pasta	1 cup plain Greek yogurt
4 cups fresh spinach	½ teaspoon onion powder
8 ounces low-fat sharp cheddar cheese	½ teaspoon garlic powder
8 ounces low-fat Monterey Jack or mozzarella	salt and pepper, to taste

1. Cook the pasta according to the package's instructions until al dente, approximately 8 minutes.

2. Save about ½ cup of the pasta water. Return the cooked macaroni to the pot and add the spinach. Stir until spinach is slightly wilted.

3. Add about ¼ cup of the reserved pasta water to the pot, and stir in the cheeses until they begin to melt.

4. Stir in the yogurt, onion powder, garlic powder, salt, and pepper, until smooth and creamy. If the consistency needs to be thinned out, stir in the remaining pasta water.

5. Remove from heat and let stand for a few minutes to allow the sauce to thicken before serving.

SHRIMP SCAMPI

This classic is so simple to make, but so elegant in presentation. The flavors are light and rich at the same time, and it's simple to substitute healthy options like whole wheat pasta to make it even better. Use a thin pasta like spaghetti, linguini, or angel hair.

Mind foods: Whole grains, olive oil, vegetables, fish, wine

Yield: 4 to 6 servings

Prep time: 15 minutes   **Cook time:** 10 minutes

1 pound whole wheat pasta

1 tablespoon grapeseed oil

2 teaspoons olive oil

1 shallot, diced

4 cloves garlic, minced

1 pound raw shrimp, peeled, deveined, tails removed

½ teaspoon crushed red pepper flakes

¼ cup chicken or fish stock

3 tablespoons white wine

1 lemon

2 tablespoons fresh parsley

salt and pepper, to taste

1. Cook pasta according to package instructions until al dente. Drain, but reserve ½ cup of pasta water.

2. Heat the grapeseed oil in a large sauté pan over medium-high heat. Add the shallot and garlic and sauté for 2 minutes, stirring occasionally.

3. Pat the shrimp dry, then add it to the sauté pan. Immediately season with crushed red pepper flakes, salt, and pepper. Continue sautéing the shrimp with the garlic for about 3 to 4 minutes, or until cooked through. The shrimp will turn opaque and pinkish white—if translucent, it means the shrimp is still raw; if too white, it's overcooked.

4. Zest half of the lemon. Set aside. Juice the entire lemon and set aside.

5. Add the chicken or fish stock, wine, lemon juice, and lemon zest. Add pasta water if the consistency is too thick. Stir to combine and continue cooking for an additional minute or so, and then remove from heat.

6. Serve over pasta. Drizzle with olive oil and top with sprinkled parsley.

BLACK SESAME TUNA STEAK

Full of protein and healthy omega-3 fatty acids, tuna steak is not only delicious, it's good for your brain function. I prefer mine just lightly seared, but you can cook it to whatever temperature you like. Try it with some wasabi paste if you're feeling spicy.

Mind food: Fish

Yield: 4 servings

Prep time: 10 minutes   **Cook time:** 4 to 8 minutes

¼ cup low-sodium soy sauce

1 tablespoon mirin

1 tablespoon local honey

2 tablespoons sesame oil

1 tablespoon apple cider vinegar

4 tuna steaks

½ cup black sesame seeds

cooking spray

1. In a medium deep bowl, combine the soy sauce, mirin, honey, sesame oil, and apple cider vinegar.

2. Spread the sesame seeds out on a plate. Dip the tuna steaks into the soy sauce mixture, making sure to submerge them completely, but briefly: for a maximum of 2 seconds per side. Season the tuna steaks with salt and pepper and then coat them in the sesame seeds on both sides.

3. Coat a large skillet with cooking spray and heat over high heat. Place the tuna steaks on the surface and sear for about 2 minutes on each side for a medium-rare tuna steak and up to 4 minutes per side for a medium-well to well-done tuna steak. You can cook them longer if you would like them more well done.

GRILLED SALMON

I first taught my dad how to make salmon using this simple recipe. Even though it is super easy, it delivers on complex flavors. Salmon is also a great way to get protein and omega-3s. Enjoy this with a side Strawberry Spinach Salad (page 71) or Orangey Asparagus (page 133).

Mind food: Fish

Yield: 4 servings

Prep time: 10 minutes   **Cook time:** 10 minutes

4 salmon filets

1 teaspoon ground cumin

1 teaspoon ground paprika

1 teaspoon ground onion powder

1 teaspoon ground chili powder, or to taste

1 teaspoon garlic powder

salt and pepper to taste

1. Season salmon lightly with salt and pepper.

2. In a small bowl, mix the cumin, paprika, onion powder, chili powder, and garlic powder.

3. If grilling, preheat the grill to medium-high, or if using an oven, preheat to 375°F.

4. Rub spice mixture onto the salmon, and then grill or bake, skin side down, for about 10 minutes, for a medium cooked filet, or cook for longer until cooked through to desired temperature. Cooked salmon should be opaque and medium pink in color.

SWEET SOY SALMON

The sweet honey and soy sauce pairs well with the salmon, which is full of protein and omega-3s. Try it with the Sautéed Bok Choy (page 140).

Mind food: Fish

Yield: 4 servings

Prep time: 10 minutes   **Cook time:** 15 minutes

1 tablespoons honey

2 teaspoons low-sodium soy sauce

4 salmon filets

½ teaspoon sesame oil

1. Preheat the oven to 400°F.

2. Mix the honey and soy sauce in a small bowl. In a small saucepan, bring the mixture to a simmer over low to medium heat. Remove from heat once it begins to simmer.

3. Rub the salmon with the sesame oil. Brush the salmon thoroughly with the honey–soy sauce mixture. Bake, skin side down, for 15 minutes, or until cooked through. Salmon should be opaque and medium pink in color.

SLOW COOKER SPAGHETTI SQUASH

Enjoy the taste and texture of spaghetti, without the calories and simple carbohydrates. Spaghetti squash is loaded with B vitamins, which can help you feel calmer and clearer, as well as help your brain transfer memory from one area to the other. Serve this with the Bean "Meat" Balls (page 116) for a healthy, delicious vegetarian meal.

Mind foods: Vegetables, olive oil

Yield: 2 servings

Prep time: 5 minutes   **Cook time:** 4 to 6 hours

1 spaghetti squash	1 teaspoon dried basil
2 cups water	salt and pepper, to taste
2 tablespoons olive oil	

1. Carefully cut the spaghetti squash in half length-wise and place it in the slow cooker. Add water. Squash should be halfway submerged in the water.

2. Cook on medium to medium-high for 4 to 6 hours, or on low for 8 to 10 hours. Remove the squash from heat and let it cool until safe to the touch.

3. Using a spoon or fork, scoop the seeds from the cavity and discard them.

4. Using a fork, shred the inside of the squash like spaghetti strands. Season with olive oil, basil, salt, and pepper to taste.

VEGETABLE GREEN CURRY

Vegetable Green Curry is a flavorful and filling vegetarian meal. For those of you who think curry is too spicy or are intimidated by a new cuisine, this recipe can be made mild, as demonstrated below, or you can make it medium or spicy by adding more spices. It's very simple to make. You can add chicken to this dish for more protein, if you'd like.

MIND foods: Whole grains, vegetables, leafy green vegetables

Yield: 4 servings

Prep time: 5 minutes   **Cook time:** 30 minutes

1 cup uncooked brown rice

water, as needed

1 tablespoon grapeseed oil

1 small yellow onion, diced

1 tablespoon minced fresh ginger

4 cloves garlic, minced

10 stalks green asparagus, chopped into 2-inch segments, ends removed

3 medium carrots, peeled and chopped

2 tablespoons Thai green curry paste

1 (14-ounce) can light coconut milk

1 teaspoon honey

2 cups spinach

fresh cilantro

crushed red pepper flakes, to taste

1. Cook the brown rice as the package instructions direct, but with a at least a cup more water than needed. After about 40 minutes, remove from heat and drain most of the water, retaining about a cup of water from the rice. Return the rice to pot. Cover and let it rest.

2. Heat 1 tablespoon of grapeseed oil in a large, deep skillet over medium heat. Sauté the onion, ginger, and garlic for 2 to 3 minutes. Add the asparagus and carrots and cook for 3 minutes, stirring often. Add the curry paste and cook, stirring often, for 2 more minutes.

3. Add the coconut milk into the pan, along with the honey and ½ cup of the water from the rice. Bring the pan to a simmer. Cook until the carrots are tender, about 10 more minutes. Add more rice water as needed to thin out the mixture.

4. Add the spinach into the mixture and cook about 30 more seconds. Remove the curry from heat and season lightly with fresh cilantro and crushed red pepper flakes.

QUINOA RISOTTO

I worked in an Italian restaurant for several years. Their risotto was to die for, but it was also stick-to-your-ribs heavy. By using quinoa, this recipe offers a lighter dish, a complete protein, and a beautiful, delicious meal.

Mind foods: Whole grains, olive oil, vegetables

Yield: 4 to 6 servings

Prep time: 15 minutes **Cook time:** 25 minutes

1½ cups quinoa, rinsed

½ cup panko bread crumbs

2 tablespoons olive oil

1½ teaspoons dried rosemary, divided

3 cloves garlic, minced

4 large tomatoes (such as Beefsteak, Heirloom, or Big Boy), halved and seeded

1 lemon

2 tablespoons grapeseed oil

1 large shallot, finely chopped

2 cups low-sodium chicken stock

Vegan Parmesan "Cheese" (page 170), low-fat cheese, or nutritional yeast, to taste

fresh parsley, to taste

salt and pepper, to taste

1. Preheat the oven to 375°F.

2. Cook the quinoa as directed, and then let it stand, covered, for about 15 minutes.

3. While the quinoa stands, use a medium bowl to mix the panko bread crumbs with the olive oil, ½ teaspoon of the rosemary, half of the garlic, and a pinch of pepper.

4. On a baking sheet, place the tomatoes with their cut sides up and top with the panko bread crumb mixture. Bake for 25 minutes, or until the crumbs are lightly browned and the tomatoes are softened. Keep warm covered with foil.

5. Zest the lemon, saving 1 teaspoon zest. Set aside. Cut the fruit into ¼-inch sections.

6. In a medium pot, heat the grapeseed oil over medium heat. Add the shallot and remaining garlic and cook, stirring, until the shallot is softened but the garlic is not burnt. Add the remaining rosemary and cook for 1 more minute. Remove from heat.

7. Add stock to the standing quinoa and bring to a boil. Reduce to a simmer over medium heat, stirring until the quinoa seems thick and viscous.

8. Remove from heat and add lemon zest, lemon sections, and the cheese or nutritional yeast. Season with pepper and parsley to taste. Serve the risotto in bowls and top with the baked tomatoes.

TANGY BRUSSELS SPROUTS PASTA

Brussels sprouts in pasta may not seem like a natural choice, and, indeed, this dish was born of my family's Leftover Night—and it works. Brussels sprouts have tons of brain-health nutrients, including vitamins K and C. They also have tryptophan, an essential amino acid, and even omega-3 fatty acids. For this dish, use a pasta like rotini, penne, or rigatoni.

Mind foods: Vegetables, olive oil, whole grains

Yield: 4 servings

Prep time: 20 minutes   **Cook time:** 40 minutes

½ pound Brussels sprouts, cut into quarters or halves

4 tablespoons olive oil, divided

½ teaspoon crushed red pepper flakes

8 ounces whole grain pasta

1 tablespoon grainy mustard

1 to 2 tablespoons local honey

Vegan Parmesan "Cheese" (page 170) or low-fat cheese, as desired for topping

1. Preheat the oven to 450°F.

2. In a bowl, toss the Brussels sprouts with 2 tablespoons of olive oil and the crushed red pepper flakes, then spread them in a single layer on a baking sheet. Roast for 30 to 40 minutes until browned.

3. While the Brussels sprouts are cooking, cook the pasta according to package directions, boiling it for about 8 minutes to be slightly al dente. Reserve 1 cup of pasta water to the side after the pasta is drained.

4. Return pasta to the pot and add remaining 2 tablespoons olive oil and mustard. Stir until well combined. Add enough of the pasta water to make a light sauce.

5. When the Brussels sprouts have finished cooking, add them to the pasta mixture and gently toss.

6. Drizzle honey over the pasta mixture and then toss until combined. Top with cheese as desired.

CASHEW CHICKEN STIR-FRY

Stir-fry is a quick and easy dish that can be made healthy and MIND-diet–friendly with a few simple adjustments. This can be eaten as is, or with a side of steamed brown rice.

Mind foods: Poultry, vegetables, wine, nuts

Yield: 4 to 6 servings

Prep time: 10 minutes   **Cook time:** 20 minutes

1½ pounds boneless, skinless chicken breasts cut into thin strips

¼ teaspoon salt

½ teaspoon pepper

4 teaspoons cornstarch

1 tablespoon grapeseed oil

2 cloves garlic, minced

2 teaspoons minced fresh ginger

1 red, orange, or yellow bell pepper, chopped

1½ cups chopped broccoli

1 cup chopped raw cashews

⅓ cup white wine

1 serving Low-Sodium Stir-Fry Sauce (page 164)

¼ cup finely chopped green onions, for garnish

1. In a large bowl, combine chicken strips, salt, pepper, and 2 teaspoons of cornstarch. Make sure that the chicken is thoroughly coated.

2. Over medium-high heat, heat 1 tablespoon of grapeseed oil in a large skillet. Cook the chicken for 5 to 6 minutes, flipping halfway through.

3. Add the garlic and ginger, and sauté for 1 minute, stirring often.

4. Add bell pepper, broccoli, and cashews, and cook for 2 to 3 more minutes.

5. Add wine to the mixture and stir well to combine. Reduce the heat to medium-low.

6. Add Low-Sodium Stir-Fry sauce and stir well to combine. Cook for 10 more minutes.

7. If sauce isn't thick enough, add the remaining cornstarch a bit at a time until the sauce reaches the desired consistency.

8. Top with green onions and serve.

HERBED RAINBOW TROUT

This fish has a nice, subtle flavor that is a little bit like salmon, but it can be easily overpowered, so treat it simply with some tomatoes, garlic, and lemon, as suggested here. And don't be afraid to try new things!

Mind foods: Fish, vegetables

Yield: 4 servings

Prep time: 15 minutes **Cook time:** 15 minutes

4 rainbow trout filets

2 large tomatoes, peeled, seeded, and chopped

4 cloves garlic, sliced thinly

1 teaspoon grapeseed oil

1 tablespoon dried thyme

1 teaspoon dried rosemary

1 lemon, sliced into quarters

handful of chopped fresh parsley, to garnish

salt and pepper, to taste

1. Preheat the oven to 450°F.

2. Season the trout on both sides with salt and pepper and then place the trout, skin side down, on the baking dish.

3. In a medium bowl, combine the tomatoes, garlic, and 1 teaspoon grapeseed oil. Spoon the mixture over the middle of each piece of trout. Season with thyme and rosemary.

4. Bake for 10 to 15 minutes. Serve with lemon wedges and parsley.

CHICKEN PARMESAN

Chicken Parmesan can be made into a MIND-diet–healthy dish with a few simple adjustments: Serve with whole grain pasta or a side of Broccoli Rabe Sauté (page 141).

Mind foods: Whole grains, poultry

Yield: 4 servings

Prep time: 10 minutes   **Cook time:** 15 minutes

2 eggs

½ cup whole wheat flour

1 tablespoon onion powder

1 tablespoon garlic powder

1 tablespoon Italian seasoning

1 tablespoon grapeseed oil

4 boneless, skinless chicken breasts

1 cup Marinara Sauce (page 157)

4 slices vegan or low-fat mozzarella cheese

salt and pepper, to taste

1. Crack the eggs in a medium, deep bowl and whisk together.

2. Mix the flour, onion powder, garlic powder, and Italian seasoning together in a separate medium, deep bowl.

3. Coat a large skillet with the oil and heat over medium.

4. Pat the chicken breasts dry, and then, one at a time, dip each one in the egg mixture and then into the flour and spice mixture, making sure to coat evenly. Immediately place the chicken in the skillet and cook for 4 to 5 minutes on each side.

5. Place the chicken on a baking sheet. Top each piece with ¼ cup of Marinara Sauce, and place a slice of mozzarella in the center of each piece.

6. Turn the oven on to a low broil, and broil the chicken just until the cheese melts. Broiler temperatures differ, so keep an eye on it: it could take 30 seconds to 1 minute.

7. Season with salt and pepper, to taste.

BAKED FISH 'N' SWEET CHIPS

My husband grew up in Australia, and fish and chips was one of his favorite dishes. This take on the classic dish is baked, not fried, and uses sweet potatoes instead of classic white potatoes. Sweet potatoes are high in vitamin A, an antioxidant that helps regulate the repair and growth systems in our bodies.

Mind foods: Vegetables, olive oil, whole grains, fish

Yield: 4 servings

Prep time: 20 minutes   **Cook time:** 25 minutes

2 large sweet potatoes, sliced into chips	1¼ cups panko bread crumbs
¼ cup extra-virgin olive oil	⅓ cup whole wheat flour
1 teaspoon garlic powder	2 large eggs
2 tablespoons fresh rosemary leaves	1½ pounds skinless cod filet, cut into 1-inch-thick strips
	salt and pepper, to taste

1. Preheat oven to 450°F.

2. Soak the potatoes in very warm water for 5 minutes, then drain and pat dry.

3. Place the potatoes in a medium bowl. Toss the chips with oil, garlic powder, and rosemary. Season with salt and pepper, to taste, and spread on a baking sheet.

4. Bake for 20 minutes, or until the potatoes reach the desired level of crispiness.

5. On a separate rack, toast the panko bread crumbs for about 5 minutes. Transfer to a medium dish.

6. Place the flour in a different medium dish and season with salt and pepper. In a third medium dish, whisk the eggs together.

7. Season the fish with salt and pepper on both sides. Then coat it in the flour, then dip it in the eggs, and then roll it in panko.

8. Finally, place the fish on a baking sheet. Bake for 15 to 18 minutes. The fish will be cooked when the center is white and flaky, and not translucent.

BAKED MACKEREL

Mackerel is excellent for brain health, providing about 600 percent of the daily recommended intake of omega-3 fatty acids, which may help prevent cognitive decline. You can cook it, and eat it, like a steak—finish this in the broiler for the last minute or so.

Mind food: Fish

Yield: 2 servings

Prep time: 5 minutes **Cook time:** 22 minutes

2 mackerel filets, skin on	½ lemon, cut into wedges
½ teaspoon grapeseed oil	salt and pepper, to taste

1. Preheat the oven to 350°F.

2. Brush the mackerel lightly with oil and then season with salt and pepper.

3. Place the mackerel in the oven and bake for about 20 minutes, until the center is opaque. Broil for another minute or two to crisp it up.

4. Sprinkle with lemon juice and serve.

SOLE AMANDINE

Sole is an incredibly mild and light fish. It will please even the people in your life who claim to not like fish; they just haven't tried it this way. My mom used to make this almond crumble for our fish. Along with the omega-3s present in the sole, almonds also contain omega-3s and are loaded with vitamin B6, which helps promote brain health, and vitamin E, which helps slow down the aging of brain cells that impact memory. The magnesium in almonds helps strengthen the nerves in the brain.

Mind foods: Nuts, fish

Yield: 2 servings

Prep time: 5 minutes   **Cook time:** 10 minutes

3 teaspoons grapeseed oil, divided

¼ cup slivered raw almonds

2 sole filets

1 lemon, juiced

salt and pepper, to taste

1. Heat 1 teaspoon grapeseed oil over medium-high heat in a skillet. Add the slivered almonds and cook for 2 to 3 minutes to toast, being extra careful not to burn them. Remove from heat and set aside, keeping warm, if possible.

2. Season the sole with salt and pepper, to taste. Wipe the skillet clean and add the remaining 2 teaspoons oil.

3. Over medium-high heat, cook the sole filets for 2 to 3 minutes on each side. Lower the heat to medium-low and add the lemon juice.

4. Cover and cook for another 3 minutes, until fish is cooked through. The center of the fish should be opaque.

5. Remove from heat and sprinkle the fish with the almonds.

BEAN "MEAT" BALLS

Eight years of being a vegan makes a person become very inventive. Luckily, these "meat" balls have been perfected and have never let me down. They pair well with whole grain pasta or with the Slow Cooker Spaghetti Squash (page 101). For a vegan alternative, use low-sodium soy sauce instead of the Worcestershire sauce.

Mind foods: Beans, vegetables, whole grains, nuts

Yield: 4 to 6 servings

Prep time: 10 minutes   **Cook time:** 20 minutes

2 (15-ounce) cans low-sodium kidney beans, rinsed and drained

3 tablespoons grapeseed oil, divided

1 medium yellow onion, chopped

1 teaspoon garlic powder

2 teaspoons dried oregano

2 teaspoons dried basil

2 tablespoons tomato paste

2 teaspoons low-sodium Worcestershire sauce

1 cup steel cut oats

⅔ cup sunflower seeds

salt and pepper, to taste

1. In a medium bowl, mash the kidney beans with a fork until they are like a thick paste.

2. In a medium skillet, heat 1 tablespoon of grapeseed oil and sauté the onion for 3 minutes. Remove from heat.

3. Add the sautéed onion to the mashed beans together with the garlic powder, oregano, basil, tomato paste, Worcestershire sauce, and oats.

4. In a food processor or high speed blender, pulse the sunflower seeds until a fine meal is achieved.

5. Add the sunflower seeds to the bean mixture and combine well. Season with salt and pepper to taste. Form 24 to 30 balls.

6. Cook the bean balls in batches: In a large pan, heat the remaining oil over medium heat and gently cook the bean balls until they are golden brown, turning them to brown on all sides, about 5 to 7 minutes.

SWEET POTATO AND ASPARAGUS HASH

This is another recipe born of my family's Leftover Night: How can we make an amazing, healthy meal out of what we have in the pantry? I encourage you to be creative and use ingredients that you like. Add or subtract to your taste. Serve each portion with a soft-boiled or over-easy egg for a heartier meal. Asparagus is full of B vitamins, folate, and vitamin A, all of which help promote brain health. One cup of asparagus provides 180 percent of the daily recommended amount of vitamin K, which helps regulate calcium in the bones and in the brain.

Mind foods: Poultry, vegetables

Yield: 4 servings

Prep time: 10 minutes   **Cook time:** 25 minutes

1 pound boneless, skinless chicken breasts	½ teaspoon crushed red pepper flakes
1 tablespoons grapeseed oil	½ bunch asparagus, cut into 2-inch chunks, ends trimmed
3 cloves garlic, minced	
1 medium sweet potato, peeled and diced	¼ teaspoon chili powder
	salt and pepper, to taste
½ cup water	

1. Season the chicken with salt and pepper.

2. Over medium heat, heat the oil. Add the chicken. Cook for 5 minutes, then flip the chicken and cook for 5 minutes more. Add the garlic when you flip the chicken.

3. Cut the chicken into bite sized pieces and set aside.

4. In the same skillet, add the sweet potato and water. Season the sweet potato with the crushed red pepper flakes.

5. Cook for about 10 minutes or until the sweet potato is tender.

6. Add the asparagus and season with chili powder. Sauté for about 5 minutes. Add the chicken and stir well to combine. Cook for another 2 minutes.

7. Remove from heat and serve.

HEARTY VEGETABLE RIGATONI

This pasta dish is chock full of fresh vegetables and seasoning, and extremely light while still warm and hearty.

Mind foods: Whole grains, vegetables, olive oil
Yield: 4 to 6 servings
Prep time: 10 minutes   **Cook time:** 30 minutes

1 pound whole wheat rigatoni	½ teaspoon garlic powder
2 green zucchini, sliced into thin discs	3 tablespoons olive oil, divided
1 eggplant, peeled and sliced thinly	3 cups Marinara Sauce (page 157)
1 teaspoon dried basil	¼ cup fresh parsley, chopped
½ teaspoon dried oregano	salt and pepper, to taste

1. Cook pasta according to package directions until it's al dente, about 8 minutes. Drain pasta, but reserve ½ cup of pasta water.

2. Preheat the oven to 450°F. In a medium bowl, combine the zucchini and eggplant and season with salt, pepper, basil, oregano, and garlic powder. Coat with 2 tablespoons of the olive oil.

3. Spread the zucchini and eggplant slices evenly on a baking sheet and bake for 15 to 20 minutes, or until browned. Remove from heat.

4. Add pasta back to the pot. Add vegetables. Stir well to combine.

5. Add salt and pepper to taste. Drizzle with remaining oil and sprinkle with parsley and serve.

ROSEMARY CHICKEN SKILLET

If you don't own a cast iron skillet, I highly recommend one. We got ours at a discount home shop for $11. If you season it well, you can use these as a non-chemical alternative to nonstick pans, and you'll consume less fat from oils as well. This recipe works great in a cast iron skillet. Rosemary, used fresh here if possible, is a brain-healthy herb that may help improve memory.

Mind foods: Poultry, vegetables

Yield: 4 servings

Prep time: 10 minutes   **Cook time:** 30 minutes

¼ cup grapeseed oil

4 boneless, skinless chicken breasts

2 sweet potatoes, chopped

2 tablespoons fresh rosemary

2 lemons

6 cloves garlic, minced

salt and pepper, to taste

1. Preheat the oven to 400°F.

2. Add grapeseed oil to a large cast iron skillet and heat over medium-high.

3. Season the chicken with salt and pepper and add to the skillet. Add the sweet potatoes. Season with rosemary and stir well to combine.

4. Cook for 5 minutes, stirring the sweet potatoes occasionally.

5. Juice 1 lemon. Pour the lemon juice and garlic over the chicken and potatoes. Flip the chicken, and cook for 5 minutes more, stirring occasionally.

6. Slice the remaining lemon and place the slices on top of the chicken. Bake for 20 minutes, or until the chicken is cooked through.

7. Remove from heat and serve.

TURKEY BOLOGNESE

Bolognese sauce is one of my family's long-time favorites. We had Italian family members, so this sauce often made an appearance at family events. Using turkey and whole grain pasta is a great way to make healthy choices for a favorite, classic dish. Pastas like rigatoni, rotini, and penne work best with this recipe.

Mind foods: Whole grains, vegetables, poultry

Yield: 4 servings

Prep time: 10 minutes **Cook time:** 30 minutes

1 pound whole grain pasta

1 tablespoon grapeseed oil

1 large sweet yellow onion, chopped

1 large carrot, peeled and chopped

1 stalk of celery, chopped

3 cloves garlic, minced

1 pound lean ground turkey

2 (15-ounce) cans low-sodium crushed tomatoes

½ cup red wine

¼ cup fresh parsley, chopped and divided

2 teaspoons dried oregano

Vegan Parmesan "Cheese" (page 170) or low-fat Parmesan

salt and pepper, to taste

1. Cook pasta according to package directions until it's al dente, about 8 minutes. Drain pasta, but reserve ½ cup of pasta water. Return pasta to pot.

2. While the pasta cooks, heat oil over medium heat in a large pan. Add onion, carrot, and celery and cook for 3 minutes. Add garlic and cook another 3 to 4 minutes.

3. Add ground turkey and cook for about 4 to 5 minutes.

4. Add the crushed tomatoes, wine, half the parsley, and oregano. Season to taste with salt and pepper.

5. Turn the heat down to medium low. Let the mixture simmer, adding pasta water as needed, for 10 to 15 minutes.

6. Add the Bolognese sauce to the pasta pot and stir gently to combine.

7. Serve sprinkled with remaining parsley and the cheese. Season with salt and pepper as needed.

CREAMY CHICKEN ALFREDO

Alfredo is so creamy and luxurious. It's pretty to look at, with the little green pops of color, and it's delicious to eat. For a MIND Diet version, I use nondairy milk and low-fat Greek yogurt and low-fat cheese for healthier substitutes from the original recipe. Long pastas like linguine, fettuccine, and spaghetti work best with this recipe.

Mind foods: Whole grains, poultry, vegetables

Yield: 4 servings

Prep time: 15 minutes   **Cook time:** 40 minutes

1 pound whole grain pasta

4 tablespoons grapeseed oil, divided

2 boneless, skinless chicken breasts

2 cloves garlic, minced

2 tablespoons whole wheat flour

¾ cup unsweetened nondairy milk

⅔ cup vegan or low-fat Parmesan cheese

½ cup low-fat Greek yogurt

1 cup peas (canned or frozen—if canned, drain and rinse well)

handful fresh parsley, chopped

salt and pepper, to taste

1. Cook pasta according to package directions until it's al dente, about 8 minutes. Drain pasta and reserve ½ cup of pasta water. Return pasta to pot.

2. Season the chicken with salt and pepper. In a large skillet over medium heat, heat 2 tablespoons oil, then add the chicken. Cook for about 5 minutes per side, or until cooked through. Chicken should be white and opaque throughout. Remove from heat and let cool, then chop into bite-sized pieces.

3. Wipe out the skillet. Return the skillet to medium-low heat and heat the remaining 2 tablespoons grapeseed oil. Add the garlic and cook for about 2 minutes. Add the flour and cook for 2 minutes more, stirring constantly, and keeping the mixture from sticking to the bottom of the skillet.

4. Slowly whisk in the milk and reduce the heat to medium low. Let the mixture simmer, stirring gently, then add the cheese and whisk until smooth. Use pasta water to thin sauce if needed.

5. Turn off the heat and whisk in Greek yogurt.

6. Pour the sauce into the pasta pot and add the chopped chicken. Stir to combine. Bring the peas to at least room temperature, then gently food them in to the pasta mixture. Serve sprinkled with parsley.

KUNG PAO TOFU AND BROCCOLI

This dish is a MIND-Diet–friendly spin on Kung Pao, using Low-Sodium Kung Pao Sauce (page 165) and unsalted peanuts. Broccoli contains vitamin K, which helps regulate calcium in the bones and the brain; choline, which helps improve memory; and folate, which is crucial for brain function. This dish is delicious on its own or served with steamed brown rice.

Mind foods: Vegetables, nuts

Yield: 4 servings

Prep time: 1 hour   **Cook time:** 25 minutes

1 block extra firm tofu

1 tablespoon grapeseed oil

½ cup water

2 large broccoli crowns, chopped

½ teaspoon chili powder

½ teaspoon crushed red pepper flakes

1 recipe Low-Sodium Kung Pao Sauce (page 165)

½ cup unsalted peanuts, chopped

3 green onions, sliced thinly

salt and pepper, to taste

1. Drain the tofu and pat dry. Season with salt and pepper. Using a sharp knife, gently press down on the top of the tofu and carefully slice horizontally through the center, so that you have 2 thinner blocks. From there, slice the tofu into bite-sized cubes. Place the tofu in an airtight container and freeze for at least an hour. The longer you freeze it, the crispier it will be when you cook it.

2. Remove from the freezer once you're ready to cook.

3. In a large pan, heat the grapeseed oil over medium-high heat. Add the tofu and cook, using a wooden spatula or spoon to break the tofu cubes gently apart. Stir occasionally and let the tofu brown on all sides, about 10 minutes.

4. Remove the tofu from the heat and set aside in a small bowl.

5. In the same pan, add the water and the broccoli. Cover and cook over medium-high heat for 5 to 10 minutes, or until the broccoli is bright green. Add the tofu back to the pan and stir to combine. Season with chili powder and red pepper and stir.

6. Add the Low-Sodium Kung Pao Sauce and stir well to combine. Cook for 5 minutes, stirring occasionally, or until the sauce is well incorporated.

7. Remove from heat. Serve with sliced green onions and chopped peanuts.

BROCCOLI RABE ORECCHIETTE

The Italian restaurant I worked at for years made a version of this dish. Orecchiette isn't a common shape of pasta, but it always tickled me a little bit to see: It looks like little ears. This dish is spicy and flavorful, and chicken sausage packs all of the delicious flavors of pork sausage with much less fat and sodium. If whole wheat orecchiette pasta is unavailable, try penne or another small shaped pasta.

Mind foods: Whole grains, leafy green vegetables, poultry, olive oil

Yield: 4 to 6 servings

Prep time: 10 minutes   **Cook time:** 30 minutes

1 pound whole wheat orecchiette pasta

3 tablespoons grapeseed oil, divided

2 cloves garlic

¼ teaspoon crushed red pepper flakes

2 bunches broccoli rabe, chopped, stems removed

4 hot Italian-style nitrate-free chicken sausage links, sliced into ½-inch pieces

½ teaspoon onion powder

1 tablespoon olive oil

salt and pepper, to taste

½ teaspoon fresh basil

1. Cook the pasta according to the package's instructions until al dente, approximately 8 minutes. Drain and reserve ½ cup of pasta water. Return the pasta to the pot.

2. Coat a large pan with 2 tablespoons grapeseed oil and heat over medium-high. Add the garlic and red pepper and cook for 2 minutes, stirring frequently. Add the broccoli rabe and stir well, making sure it's coated in the garlic and red pepper.

3. Add water, as needed, to help the broccoli rabe cook down, stirring frequently. Cook for 5 to 7 minutes, or until broccoli rabe is tender but still bright green. Remove from heat.

4. Add the broccoli rabe to the pasta pot.

5. Wipe out the skillet and add the remaining tablespoon of grapeseed oil. Add the sausage and cook until it's no longer pink in the center, stirring occasionally, about 10 minutes.

6. Add the sausage to the pasta pot. Turn to medium-low heat and stir well, adding the onion powder. Add pasta water, a little at a time, as you stir. Cook for 3 to 5 more minutes until the mixture is well combined and slightly thickened.

7. Remove the pasta mixture from the heat. Drizzle with olive oil, season with salt and pepper, and sprinkle with basil.

COLORFUL GUMBO

The cuisine of New Orleans had a big effect on me. It's so flavorful and rich, but can be very unhealthy. I firmly believe in enjoying food, so it was my personal mission to make as many recipes from my experience there into healthy dishes I could enjoy at home. Enjoy this colorful version with brown rice or quinoa. Note: Creating a roux is much less intimidating than it seems, and actually pretty fun to do!

Mind foods: Whole grains, vegetables, fish, leafy greens

Yield: 4 to 6 servings

Prep time: 10 minutes   **Cook time:** 45 minutes

3 tablespoons grapeseed oil

3 tablespoons whole wheat flour

½ medium sweet yellow onion, chopped

1 green bell pepper, seeded and chopped

1 yellow bell pepper, seeded and chopped

1 bay leaf

2 cloves garlic, minced

1 (8-ounce) can low or no sodium diced tomatoes

½ tablespoon paprika

½ teaspoon oregano

1 tablespoon chili powder

1½ cups water

1 pound raw shrimp, peeled, deveined, tails removed

1 cup kale, chopped, ribs removed

2 tablespoons parsley

salt and pepper, to taste

1. Create a roux by whisking the grapeseed oil and the flour together in a pan over medium heat, being careful to not let it burn or stick. Continue to mix with a wooden spoon or flat spatula, scraping the sides and the bottom of the pan, for about 15 to 20 minutes, or until the roux turns a dark caramel color.

2. Add the onion, peppers, bay leaf, garlic, and tomatoes to the roux. Season with the paprika, oregano, and chili powder. Sauté for 5 to 7 minutes or until the vegetables begin to soften. If the mixture becomes too thick, add a few tablespoons of water.

3. Add the water and stir well to combine. Cook for 2 to 3 more minutes, or until the mixture begins to simmer.

4. Reduce the heat to medium low and add the shrimp. Stir well and cook for about 10 more minutes, stirring occasionally. Shrimp will be done when whitish pink and opaque—if translucent, it means the shrimp is still raw; if too white, it's overcooked.

5. Add the kale and stir gently to combine. Cook for 2 more minutes, until kale is just cooked.

6. Remove from heat. Remove the bay leaf, sprinkle with parsley, and serve.

CHAPTER 5
SIDES

A side dish should be a perfect complement to your main. Think bigger than boring baked potatoes or simple side salads. Your side should be fun and flavorful. It should help bring out the flavors of and add to the overall experience of the main dish, not take away from it with overwhelming textures or too much strong spice of its own. Think about how you want to accentuate your main dish: which textures, flavors, and even temperatures? Do you want something warm, like sweet potato fries? Or something cool and refreshing, like slaw?

Mind–Body Tip: Try to sleep for at least 7 hours to give your body and brain time to restore.

ORANGEY ASPARAGUS

Orange adds bright, citrusy notes to this asparagus, while the walnuts make it crunchy and interesting. This pairs well with the Grilled Salmon (page 99).

Mind foods: Nuts, vegetables, olive oil

Yield: 4 servings

Prep time: 15 minutes **Cook time:** 15 minutes

1 orange, juiced and zested

½ cup walnuts

¼ teaspoon crushed red pepper flakes

4 cups water

1 bunch asparagus, ends trimmed

2 tablespoons olive oil

salt and pepper, to taste

1. In a small pot, bring the juice from the orange to a boil over medium-high heat. Reduce to medium-low and simmer for 10 minutes. Remove from heat and set aside.

2. Preheat the oven to 375°F. Spread the walnuts in a single layer on a baking sheet, sprinkle with red pepper, and bake. Start checking on the walnuts after about 5 minutes to ensure they don't burn. They will be done between 5 and 10 minutes.

3. Remove the walnuts from the heat and let them cool before you chop them. Set aside.

4. In a medium pot, bring water to a boil. Blanch the asparagus in boiling water for 2 to 4 minutes. Drain and rinse in cold water or in an ice bath.

5. Add the olive oil to the orange juice and whisk until well blended. Season with salt and pepper.

6. In a large bowl, toss asparagus with orange juice mixture and half of the orange zest. Sprinkle with walnut pieces and serve.

LEMON COUSCOUS

Couscous is simple to make: It takes a few minutes, and only a couple of ingredients. It also has a very mild flavor on its own, so I played with seasonings for a long time before settling on the bright notes of lemon and basil for this dish.

Mind foods: Whole grains, leafy green vegetables

Yield: 4 servings

Prep time: 5 minutes   **Cook time:** 5 minutes

1 cup couscous	2 tablespoons fresh basil
4 cups chopped spinach	salt and pepper, to taste
½ lemon, juiced and zested	

1. Cook couscous according to package instructions.

2. Remove from heat and add spinach and lemon zest, stirring to combine, for about 1 minute. Spinach should just barely wilt. Serve sprinkled with lemon juice and basil.

DAD'S FAVORITE BRUSSELS SPROUTS

I lived with my dad for a bit after graduate school, and one day I made Brussels sprouts for us. He wrinkled his nose, remembering how they had always been cooked: boiled and plain. When he tasted this recipe, he was flabbergasted: How could Brussels sprouts be so delicious? They're a common request when I visit now. Filled with vitamins K and C, as well as the essential amino acid tryptophan and omega-3s, they're great for brain health as well.

Mind food: Vegetables

Yield: 4 to 6 servings

Prep time: 10 minutes   **Cook time:** 20 minutes

2 pounds Brussels sprouts, quartered

2 tablespoons grapeseed oil

¼ cup balsamic vinegar

2 tablespoons whole grain Dijon mustard

½ teaspoon crushed red pepper flakes

½ teaspoon ground paprika

¼ teaspoon dried chili powder

½ teaspoon garlic powder

1 teaspoon dried basil

1. Preheat oven to 425°F.

2. In a large bowl, coat Brussels sprouts with grapeseed oil. Toss with vinegar and mustard, and add seasonings. Pour into a baking dish.

3. Bake for 20 minutes or until crispy, stirring once.

SUPER SLAW

Often slaw can be too heavy with dressing, or just a bunch of cabbage and iceberg lettuce smothered in mayonnaise and salt. Not this super slaw! Packed with nutrients, it may not be classic, but it's delicious.

Mind foods: Vegetables, leafy green vegetables, olive oil

Yield: 8 servings

Prep time: 20 minutes

1 head of cabbage, sliced into strips

1 bunch kale, stems removed and sliced into strips

1 bell pepper, seeded and diced

1 medium carrot, peeled and grated

2 lemons, juiced, ½ lemon zested

¼ cup extra-virgin olive oil

1 tablespoon local honey

salt and pepper, to taste

Add all ingredients in a large bowl and combine thoroughly.

SAUTÉED SWISS CHARD

I don't know how it is at your house, but in ours, we're always trying to come up with new ways to get more greens in—they're just too good for us to not have, because they are rich in vitamins we need to keep our brains healthy and our bodies strong. Swiss chard has a milder flavor than kale does, and it's easy to make. It's also packed with vitamin A and contains about three times the recommended daily intake of vitamin K. Just make sure to wash it well as it can be pretty gritty!

Mind foods: Leafy green vegetables, olive oil

Yield: 4 servings

Prep time: 10 minutes   **Cook time:** 10 minutes

2 tablespoons grapeseed oil

6 cloves garlic, sliced thinly

3 bunches well-rinsed rainbow chard, chopped, ends trimmed

½ teaspoon crushed red pepper flakes

3 tablespoons olive oil

½ lemon, juiced

salt and pepper, to taste

1. In a large pan, heat the grapeseed oil over medium heat.

2. Add the garlic and sauté for 1 minute. Add the chard and season with the red pepper. Cook for 3 minutes, stirring often.

3. Reduce heat to medium-low and cover. Cook for 3 more minutes and stir.

4. Cook until chard is tender, 1 or 2 more minutes. Remove from heat. Toss with olive oil and lemon juice. Season with salt and pepper.

SLOW COOKER COLLARD GREENS

Collard greens are one of the staples of Southern living. Often, these will be the only green food on a menu in a Southern restaurant. They will usually be cooked in lard and contain fatback or bacon. While I love collard greens, I don't love all that added fat and sodium. This recipe has all of the flavor, and much less fat and sodium than the classic version.

Mind foods: Leafy green vegetables, poultry, vegetables

Yield: 4 servings

Prep Time: 30 minutes   **Cook time:** 4 to 6 hours

4 cups low-sodium chicken stock, plus more as needed

1½ tablespoons apple cider vinegar

1½ tablespoons local honey

½ teaspoon crushed red pepper flakes

½ teaspoon ground paprika

1 pound fresh collard greens

¼ pound natural nitrate-free turkey bacon, diced

¼ medium sweet yellow onion, finely chopped

2 cloves garlic, finely minced

pepper, to taste

1. In the slow cooker, combine half the chicken stock, half the apple cider vinegar, half the honey, half the crushed red pepper flakes, and half the paprika. Cook on high while you prepare the rest.

2. Remove the stems from the collard greens and chop the leaves into 1-inch pieces. Wash them well in a colander.

3. Cook the turkey bacon in a large skillet until rendered and browned, about 8 minutes. Season with black pepper, to taste. About halfway through, add the chopped onion. Cook, stirring well, until the onion is softened, about 4 minutes.

4. Add the minced garlic to the skillet and cook for about 1 more minute. Remove the skillet from the heat.

5. Turn the slow cooker to low. Working slowly, add collards to the slow cooker, gently stirring to combine well with stock. Add the remaining chicken stock, apple cider vinegar, and honey. Add the turkey bacon, onion, and garlic mixture. Stir well.

6. Cover and cook the collards on low for 4 to 6 hours. When finished, the collards should be tender.

SAUTÉED BOK CHOY

Baby bok choy, with its tiny little heads of cabbage, seems like a story book version of cabbage—something a fairy tale character would eat. This recipe is delicious and low sodium, retaining a lot of flavor. It pairs well with the Sweet Soy Salmon (page 100).

Mind food: Leafy green vegetables

Prep time: 5 minutes   **Cook time:** 10 minutes

Yield: 4 servings

1 tablespoon grapeseed oil	1 teaspoon ground ginger
1 clove garlic, minced	1 tablespoon low-sodium soy sauce
6 small heads baby bok choy, halved lengthwise	2 tablespoons water

1. Heat the grapeseed oil in a large pan over medium-high heat.

2. Add the garlic and sauté for 30 seconds to 1 minute. Add the bok choy and season with ginger, stirring often for 1 minute. Add the soy sauce and water and cover.

3. Cook for 2 to 3 minutes. Remove the lid and continue cooking for about 2 more minutes, stirring occasionally, until the bok choy is tender.

BROCCOLI RABE SAUTÉ

Some people are intimidated by broccoli rabe because if it's not cooked correctly, it can be very bitter. This is one of my favorite vegetables, and I've learned that the trick is to break it down slowly over heat until it is soft and tender, and then drizzle it with olive oil and lemon.

Mind foods: Vegetables, leafy green vegetables, olive oil

Yield: 4 servings

Prep time: 5 minutes   **Cook time:** 10 minutes

1 tablespoon grapeseed oil	2 cups water
6 cloves garlic, sliced thinly	3 tablespoons olive oil
½ teaspoon crushed red pepper flakes	½ lemon, juiced
2 bunches broccoli rabe, chopped, stems removed	salt and pepper, to taste

1. Coat a large pan with the grapeseed oil and heat over medium-high heat.

2. Add the garlic and crushed red pepper flakes and cook for 2 minutes, stirring frequently.

3. Add the broccoli rabe and stir it well to coat in the garlic and red pepper. Add water as needed to help it cook down, stirring frequently. Cook for 5 to 7 minutes, or until the broccoli rabe is tender but still bright green.

4. Remove from heat. Season with salt and pepper and drizzle with olive oil and lemon juice.

SZECHUAN VEGETABLES

These vegetables are so quick and easy, and so packed with flavor, without the excess sodium and MSG found in many conventional Szechuan sauces. Enjoy them with Crispy Szechuan Tofu (page 90), or stir in some shrimp to soak up the delicious sauce.

Mind foods: Vegetables, leafy green vegetables, nuts

Yield: 4 servings

Prep time: 15 minutes   **Cook time:** 15 minutes

6 cups water

½ pound green beans, ends trimmed

1 tablespoon toasted sesame oil

1 red bell pepper, seeded and sliced thinly

2 cups baby bok choy, chopped

½ cup raw cashews

1 small red onion, sliced thinly

1 teaspoon low-sodium soy sauce

2 tablespoons Low-Sodium Szechuan Sauce (page 166)

1. In a medium pot, bring water to a boil. Blanch green beans in boiling water for 2 to 4 minutes. Drain and rinse the beans in cold water or an ice bath, and set aside.

2. Heat the sesame oil in a large skillet over medium-high heat. Add the green beans, red pepper, bok choy, cashews, and onion, and stir well to combine.

3. Cook, stirring occasionally, for 3 minutes. Add the soy sauce and Szechuan sauce and stir to combine.

4. Cook until the vegetables are tender, for 3 to 5 more minutes. Remove from heat.

SWEET POTATO FRIES

Sweet potatoes are full of B vitamins and fiber. This version of sweet potato fries is baked, not fried, so we like to enjoy them at least once a week.

Mind foods: Vegetables, olive oil

Yield: 2 to 4 servings

Prep time: 10 minutes **Cook time:** 30 minutes

2 sweet potatoes, sliced into ½-inch-thick wedges

1 tablespoon olive oil

½ teaspoon garlic powder

lemon juice, to taste

salt and pepper, to taste

1. Preheat oven to 450°F. Grease a baking sheet.

2. In a bowl, combine sweet potato wedges with olive oil, garlic powder, and black pepper until coated. Spread them evenly on the baking sheet.

3. Bake the sweet potato fries for about 15 minutes, and then turn them over and bake another 10 to 15 minutes until they are crispy. If you cut smaller fries, they will take less time to cook.

4. Remove from the oven and sprinkle with salt to taste. Gently squeeze lemon juice over the fries to give a light citrus flavor.

CUCUMBER AND DILL SALAD

Whenever I think of a summer picnic, I think of the cucumber salad my mother would always bring. It was refreshing and cool, and I loved how the cucumbers would crunch in my mouth. This recipe is sure to be a hit whether you enjoy it for lunch, or increase the recipe and bring it to a picnic.

Mind food: Vegetables

Yield: 2 servings

Prep time: 10 minutes

2 large cucumbers, seeded

1 small red onion, thinly sliced

1 tablespoon plus 1 teaspoon apple cider vinegar

1 teaspoon local honey

2 teaspoons dill

salt and pepper, to taste

1. Chop the cucumber into bite sized pieces.

2. In a colander, toss the cucumber and onion with the salt. Let the mixture drain for 20 minutes, then press the liquid out and rinse well with cold water.

3. In a small bowl, whisk the apple cider vinegar and honey until well combined. Dress the cucumber mixture and toss to coat. Sprinkle with dill.

CITRUS GARLIC GREEN BEANS

This dish is easy and quick to make. Blanching the green beans lets them retain their beautiful vibrant green color and crisp texture. Green beans are packed with nutrients like vitamins A, C, K, B6, and folate.

Mind foods: Vegetables, olive oil

Yield: 6 servings

Prep time: 10 minutes   **Cook time:** 10 minutes

2 pounds green beans, ends trimmed	1 teaspoon crushed red pepper flakes, to taste
1 tablespoon grapeseed oil	1 tablespoon lemon zest
2 cloves garlic, chopped	1 lemon, juiced
	1 tablespoon olive oil

1. In a large pot, blanch the green beans in boiling water for about 2 minutes. Stop when they are still bright green and crisp—don't let them overcook. Remove from heat and drain.

2. Heat a large pan over medium heat. Add grapeseed oil. Add the garlic and crushed red pepper flakes and sauté for about 1 minute. Add the beans and cook, stirring occasionally, for about 5 minutes.

3. Remove from heat. Finish with lemon zest, lemon juice, and olive oil.

HONEY-GLAZED CARROTS

When carrots are cooked, they become much sweeter—and one of my favorite vegetables. These carrots are tender and sweet. Carrots contain a compound called luteolin, which may reduce age-related inflammation in the brain, promoting better brain function.

Mind foods: Vegetables, olive oil

Yield: 4 to 6 servings

Prep time: 5 minutes   **Cook time:** 25 minutes

1 pound carrots, peeled and sliced into discs

¼ cup olive oil

2½ tablespoons honey

¼ teaspoon cumin

½ lemon, juiced

salt and pepper, to taste

1. Preheat the oven to 425°F.

2. In a medium bowl, toss carrots in olive oil, honey, and cumin.

3. In a baking dish, bake for 20 to 25 minutes, stirring once, or until carrots are tender. Remove to let cool.

4. Sprinkle with lemon juice and season with salt and pepper.

ROASTED CAULIFLOWER

Cauliflower is so fantastic because not only can it can serve as a vessel for any flavor you want, it's also full of vitamin C and contains high levels of vitamin K and folate, as well as other B vitamins. It even contains some omega-3s. I like this recipe because it combines some of my favorite seasonings into one dish.

Mind food: Vegetables

Yield: 6 to 8 servings

Prep time: 5 minutes   **Cook time:** 20 minutes

1 head cauliflower, chopped into bite-sized pieces	¼ teaspoon crushed red pepper flakes
¼ cup grapeseed oil	1 teaspoon thyme
1 teaspoon garlic powder	salt, to taste

1. Preheat the oven to 450°F.

2. In a large bowl, toss the cauliflower with the oil, garlic powder, red pepper, and thyme.

3. Spread evenly on a greased or nonstick baking sheet. Roast for 18 to 20 minutes, or until cauliflower begins to brown, stirring once halfway.

4. Remove from the oven and season with salt.

FRIED RICE

My husband loves to make this dish. It was one of the first things he made for me when we were dating. You can throw in your favorite vegetables if you want to mix things up, but these are a good base.

Mind foods: Vegetables, whole grains

Yield: 4 servings

Prep time: 15 minutes   **Cook time:** 10 minutes

2 tablespoons grapeseed oil, divided	1 medium carrot, peeled and chopped
3 green onions, thinly sliced	1 teaspoon ginger
1 clove garlic, minced	2 eggs, beaten
1 cup broccoli, chopped	2 tablespoons low-sodium soy sauce, divided
½ red bell pepper, seeded and chopped	2 cups cooked brown rice

1. In a large pan or wok, heat 1 tablespoon grapeseed oil over medium-high heat. Add the green onions and garlic and cook, stirring often, for about 30 seconds.

2. Add the vegetables and the ginger. Cook, stirring occasionally, for 3 to 4 minutes, or until mostly cooked through. Set aside.

3. In a small bowl, whisk the eggs together. Add 1 tablespoon soy sauce. Set aside.

4. Wipe out the pan. Heat 1 tablespoon grapeseed oil over medium heat. Add the cooked rice and stir often until hot, cooking for 1 to 2 minutes, scraping the bottom and the sides.

5. Add the vegetables to the mixture and stir to combine. Pour the egg mixture over the rice mixture and quickly stir, cooking the eggs into the mixture.

6. Cook for 1 to 2 more minutes, or until eggs are cooked within the mixture.

7. Remove from heat. Season with remaining soy sauce, if desired.

CAULIFLOWER RICE

Cauliflower rice is very trendy right now, as more people become aware of healthy alternatives. This recipe is flavorful and light— try it and see how it fits in to your side dish mash up.

Mind food: Vegetables

Yield: 4 servings

Prep time: 10 minutes   **Cook time:** 10 minutes

1 head cauliflower, chopped	1 clove garlic, minced
1 tablespoon grapeseed oil	2 tablespoons parsley
½ medium sweet yellow onion, chopped	½ lemon, juiced
	salt and pepper, to taste

1. Pulse the cauliflower in a food processor or a high speed blender until it's very fine and grainy, like rice.

2. Heat the grapeseed oil over medium-high heat in a large pan. Add the onion and cook, stirring often, for 3 to 4 minutes. Add the garlic and the riced cauliflower and stir to combine.

3. Cook for 3 to 5 minutes, stirring often. Remove from the heat. Sprinkle with parsley and lemon juice. Season with salt and pepper.

SAUTÉED SQUASH

In the summer, my mom would make this dish using zucchini and squash from our vegetable garden. She would cook it until it was tender and browned, and it was a sign to us that summer was here. Enjoy it with a little lemon, to make it sweet and bright.

Mind food: Vegetables

Yield: 4 to 6 servings

Prep time: 5 minutes   **Cook time:** 8 minutes

1 tablespoon grapeseed oil

1 clove garlic, minced

2 zucchini, sliced

1 summer squash, sliced

½ lemon, juiced

salt and pepper, to taste

1. Heat the grapeseed oil in a large pan over medium-high heat.

2. Add the garlic, zucchini, and squash. Cook, stirring occasionally, until the squash is tender and beginning to brown, about 7 to 8 minutes.

3. Remove from heat and sprinkle with lemon juice. Season with salt and pepper.

NUTTY SWEET RICE

When I created this dish, I was craving something crunchy and sweet, but also something that would have some weight. This recipe combines so many textures and flavors, which also means it has many vitamins and minerals. Cashews provide iron and magnesium; golden raisins contain boron, which may help improve concentration and enhance hand and eye coordination; and the brown basmati rice contains B vitamins.

Mind foods: Nuts, whole grains, vegetables

Yield: 4 to 6 servings

Prep time: 5   **Cook time:** 20 minutes

3 tablespoons raw cashews, chopped

1 cup uncooked brown basmati rice, rinsed

¼ cup naturally sweetened or low-sugar golden raisins

¼ cup naturally sweetened or low-sugar dried cranberries

2 green onions, thinly sliced

salt and pepper, to taste

1. Heat a small pan over medium-high heat and add cashews. Sauté for 1 to 2 minutes, or until lightly toasted, being careful not to burn. Set aside.

2. Cook rice according to package instructions, about 40 minutes, but do not overcook. Remove from heat and stir well.

3. Add the cashews, golden raisins, dried cranberries, salt, and pepper to the rice and stir well to combine. Place the mixture over low heat and cook for 2 to 3 minutes, stirring gently.

4. Remove from heat. Serve topped with green onions.

INDIAN-SPICED ACORN SQUASH

This acorn squash is paired with sweet, spicy flavors to bring out its natural flavors—and it, too, can be enjoyed as a side, or with the addition of some crumbled chicken sausage, as a main.

Mind food: Vegetables

Yield: 6 servings

Prep time: 15 minutes   **Cook time:** 1 hour

3 acorn squash, cut in half, seeded, pulp removed

2 tablespoons grapeseed oil

2 tablespoons local honey

1½ teaspoons curry powder

½ teaspoon ground turmeric

¼ teaspoon crushed red pepper flakes

salt and pepper, to taste

1. Preheat the oven to 375°F.

2. Drizzle the flesh of the squash with grapeseed oil and honey. Season with curry powder, turmeric, and red pepper.

3. Place on a baking sheet or in a baking dish and roast for 45 minutes to 1 hour, or until the squash is tender.

4. Remove from oven. Season with salt and pepper.

ROASTED ROOT VEGETABLES

A few years ago, we gave up on mashed, soft side dishes for Thanksgiving and started making delicious, flavorful roasted ones instead. By baking vegetables with oil and keeping the skins on, this helps the vegetables retain more nutrients. This roasted root vegetable dish is one that I enjoy year round, because I enjoy the flavors that roasting the vegetables brings out. In the summer, it pairs well with grilled fish and chicken.

Mind food: Vegetables

Yield: 4 to 6 servings

Prep time: 30 minutes   **Cook time:** 1 hour

1 butternut squash, seeded, peeled, and cubed

3 sweet potatoes, cubed

3 beets, peeled and cubed

½ small red onion, chopped

½ medium sweet yellow onion, chopped

2 tablespoons plus 1 teaspoon grapeseed oil

2 teaspoon dried thyme

2 medium carrots, peeled and chopped

⅛ teaspoon ground cumin

2 tablespoons local honey

1 head elephant garlic, cloves separated but not peeled

salt and pepper, to taste

1. Preheat the oven to 425°F.

2. In a large bowl, toss the squash, potato, beet, and onion with 2 tablespoons oil and the thyme and then pour into a baking dish.

3. Toss the carrots separately with the remaining 1 teaspoon of oil and the cumin. Add carrots to the rest of the vegetables and then add the honey. Add the garlic cloves and toss to combine.

4. Spread in an even layer on a baking sheet or in a baking dish and bake, uncovered, for 45 minutes to 1 hour, stirring once halfway. Remove from heat and season with salt and pepper.

REFRIED BEANS

This recipe takes the classic version and makes it healthy (classic versions are commonly made with lard) and is delicious with tacos, burritos, or your favorite guacamole recipe.

Mind food: Beans

Yield: 2 servings

Prep time: 5 minutes

1 (14-ounce) can low-sodium kidney, pinto, or black beans, drained and rinsed

1 teaspoon onion powder

½ teaspoon garlic powder

¼ teaspoon ground cumin

¼ teaspoon low-sodium soy sauce

red chili flakes, to taste

Combine ingredients in a food processor and pulse until smooth. Serve immediately, or, if desired, warm over low heat, stirring often, for about 5 minutes, or until just warmed.

CHAPTER 6

DIPS, DOUGHS, SAUCES, AND SEASONINGS

Ah, toppings. Extras. Dip. Dough. We don't need to sacrifice any of these things to eat a brain-healthy diet—and in fact, I think that these alternatives are more delicious because they have more flavor. White flour dough is replaced by whole grains and sunflower seeds. Peanut butter becomes honey-roasted vanilla almond butter. Plain hummus mixes with avocado or beautiful beet. The options are endless, and never boring or limiting. What will be your favorite?

Mind–Body Tip: Work on a puzzle, like a jigsaw puzzle or crossword, at some point during the day. Spending 30 to 40 minutes most days on mentally stimulating activities, like puzzles, can have brain benefits.

MARINARA SAUCE

Growing up in New Jersey meant a lot of exposure to Italian cuisine. Making Sunday sauce, or "gravy" as it was called, was practically religion. This homemade sauce is simple, and it tastes far better than anything you'll get in a jar. Eat this over whole grain pasta.

MIND foods: Vegetables; wine

Yield: 8 to 10 servings

Prep time: 10 minutes   **Cook time:** 20 minutes

1 tablespoon grapeseed oil	½ cup red wine
2 small yellow onions, chopped	2 (15-ounce) cans low-sodium diced tomatoes
4 cloves garlic, minced	2 teaspoons dried oregano
2 medium carrots, peeled and diced	2 teaspoons dried basil
2 tablespoons tomato paste	salt and pepper to taste

1. In a medium skillet, heat the oil over medium heat. Sauté the onion for 3 minutes, stirring occasionally, then add the garlic and the carrot. Cook for another 2 to 3 minutes.

2. Add the tomato paste and cook for 2 minutes. Add the red wine and allow it to evaporate before adding the diced tomatoes.

3. Let the mixture simmer for about 10 minutes. Season with oregano, basil, salt, and pepper.

SOUTHWEST DRESSING

You don't need a lot of fat and dairy to make a smooth, creamy dressing. The Greek yogurt in this dressing makes it tangy and gives you healthy probiotics. It pairs well with the Southwest Salad (page 76).

MIND food: Vegetables

Yield: 8 to 10 servings

Prep time: 10 minutes

1 avocado, diced

1 cup chopped fresh cilantro

2 cups low-fat Greek yogurt

3 green onions, chopped

3 cloves garlic, minced

1 lime, juiced

1 teaspoon local honey

Place ingredients in a food processor or high speed blender and blend until smooth. This can be stored in the refrigerator, for up to 1 week.

ROASTED GARLIC GUACAMOLE

If there is one thing I love more than roasted garlic, it's guacamole. When I created this recipe, it was all I could do not to sit and eat out of the bowl with a spoon—but no one is saying you can't. Garlic also contains vitamins, minerals, and antioxidants that help protect the body's cells against oxidative damage.

MIND foods: Fruits, olive oil

Yield: 8 to 10 servings

Prep time: 10 minutes   **Cook time:** 1 minute

cooking spray

2 cloves garlic, chopped

2 avocados, chopped, seed removed

½ small red onion, minced

1 lime, juiced

1 tablespoon extra-virgin olive oil

1 tablespoon chopped fresh cilantro

½ teaspoon crushed red pepper flakes, to taste

1. Spray a small pan with cooking spray and heat over medium heat.

2. Cook the garlic until lightly browned, about 30 seconds. Remove from heat.

3. In a medium bowl, mash the avocado until smooth. Add all ingredients to the avocado mixture and stir until blended.

BALSAMIC DIJON DRESSING

Tangy and tart, this dressing is a light compliment to your favorite salad. Pack it in an airtight container and bring it with you, or store it in the, refrigerator, for up to 2 weeks.

MIND foods: Olive oil, vegetables

Yield: 6 servings

Prep time: 2 minutes

⅓ cup olive oil

3 tablespoons balsamic vinegar

1 tablespoon local honey

1 clove garlic, minced

2 teaspoons Dijon mustard

salt and pepper, to taste

In a small bowl or jar, whisk olive oil, balsamic vinegar, honey, garlic, and Dijon mustard together until smooth and well combined. Season with salt and pepper to taste.

GARLIC SALSA

Salsa is a great dip or topping. Enjoy it with whole grain chips, on scrambled eggs or omelets, on chicken, on tacos and burritos—the options are endless. Make this recipe as spicy as you like by adding more (or less) jalapeño.

MIND food: Vegetables

Yield: 20 servings

Prep time: 10 minutes

2 (15-ounce) cans low-sodium diced tomatoes

1 green bell pepper, seeded and diced

1 small white onion, diced

2 cloves garlic, minced

¼ cup minced fresh cilantro

1 lime, juiced

1 jalapeño, diced

½ teaspoon ground cumin

salt and pepper, to taste

Combine the tomatoes, pepper, onion, garlic, cilantro, lime juice, jalapeño, cumin, and salt and pepper in a bowl.

ROASTED GARLIC

I worked in a restaurant that specialized in garlic. One of their trademarks was to serve a full head of roasted garlic with each dish. The servers would eat the roasted garlic on bread for snacks. Our breath wasn't great, but it was delicious. You can store the garlic, refrigerated for 1 week, and use it for a spread on crackers or bread, or use it to season pasta, rice, potatoes, soups, and more.

MIND foods: Vegetables, olive oil

Yield: 4 to 6 servings

Prep time: 5 minutes   **Cook time:** 40 minutes

  1 or more heads of garlic

  2 tablespoons olive oil, per head

1. Heat the oven to 400°F.

2. Peel the outer layer off the garlic as much as possible. Try to keep the head itself intact with the cloves connected.

3. Carefully cut off the very top of the head of garlic, about ¼ inch down, until the tops of the cloves garlic are exposed.

4. Place the garlic in a baking dish lined with aluminum foil with the trimmed sides facing up. Drizzle liberally with olive oil, letting the oil sink down into the cloves. Wrap the foil over until closed gently and bake for 40 minutes, or until a center clove is soft when pierced with a fork or knife.

PISTACHIO PESTO

Pesto is delicious and versatile. You can eat it on crackers, bread, in pastas, on chicken, and on salmon. This recipe is so bright and fresh, you can enjoy it however you like.

MIND foods: Vegetables, nuts, olive oil

Servings: 8

Prep time: 10 minutes

3 cups fresh basil

2 cups pistachios, shelled (optionally, toasted)

2 cloves garlic, minced

1 lemon, juiced and zested

¾ cup plus 2 tablespoons olive oil, divided

1. In food processor or high speed blender, pulse the basil, pistachios, garlic, lemon zest and juice, and 2 tablespoons olive oil.

2. While the ingredients are processing, slowly add more olive oil until it reaches desired consistency.

LOW-SODIUM STIR-FRY SAUCE

We love to make stir-fries for a quick midweek dish, but stir-fry sauce can be very high in sodium. We experimented with adaptations a lot before settling on this one—but, of course, we're always playing with levels of spice and sweet. Play with it on your own and see what tastes best for you.

MIND food: Vegetables

Yield: 4 to 6 servings

Prep time: 10 minutes   **Cook time:** 20 minutes

2 tablespoons cornstarch

¼ cup water

2 tablespoons sesame oil

2 teaspoons fresh ginger, minced

4 cloves garlic, minced

2 cups low-sodium chicken broth

¼ cup low-sodium soy sauce

¼ cup local honey

crushed red pepper flakes, to taste

1 teaspoon black pepper

1 lemon, juiced

1. In a small bowl, dissolve the cornstarch in the water and set to the side.

2. In a small saucepan, heat the sesame oil over medium heat. Add the ginger and garlic and stir-fry 15 to 30 seconds.

3. Add the chicken broth, soy sauce, honey, crushed red pepper flakes, pepper, and lemon juice. Bring to a boil, stirring. Give the cornstarch a stir, add it to the sauce, and stir to combine.

4. Over medium heat, heat until sauce thickens. Reduce heat to a simmer and cook for 30 seconds. Remove from heat and set aside. Can be frozen and used later. Reheat over low heat.

LOW-SODIUM KUNG PAO SAUCE

This American Chinese classic is one of my favorite to-go dishes, but it is usually high in MSG and sodium, which leaves me feeling a little funky. I played with this adaptation, and am always working on ways to get the spicy, sweet, garlicky, nutty flavor just right. Try this with the Kung Pao Tofu and Broccoli (page 126).

MIND food: Vegetables

Yield: 4 servings

Prep time: 5 minutes

1 cup low-sodium vegetable broth

1 tablespoon low-sodium soy sauce

3 cloves garlic, minced

1 teaspoon ginger

½ teaspoon chili powder

1 teaspoon peanut oil

¼ cup rice wine vinegar

1 tablespoon Worcestershire sauce

1½ tablespoons cornstarch

In a medium bowl, whisk all of the ingredients together. Cook with tofu, chicken, or vegetables.

LOW-SODIUM SZECHUAN SAUCE

This is the sauce to pair with your delicious fresh vegetables to make them Szechuan style, any time you want to add a (healthy) kick to your dish. There aren't any mind foods in this recipe, but it pairs fantastically with Crispy Szechuan Tofu (page 90) and Szechuan Vegetables (page 142), both of which are full of nutrients on their own.

Yield: 8

Prep time: 10 minutes   **Cook time:** 10 minutes

4 tablespoons rice wine vinegar

3 tablespoons fresh ginger, peeled and minced

6 cloves garlic, minced

1 teaspoon red pepper flakes

3 tablespoons low-sodium soy sauce

2 teaspoons local honey

½ teaspoon chili powder

1 cup water

1 tablespoon cornstarch

1. Mix rice vinegar, ginger, garlic, red pepper flakes, soy sauce, honey, and chili powder in a small pot and heat over medium-high until it is heavily simmering but not boiling.

2. While the liquid is simmering, combine the water and cornstarch in small bowl and whisk until the cornstarch is dissolved.

3. Remove the soy sauce mixture from heat and stir the cornstarch mixture in until the sauce thickens.

AVOCADO HUMMUS

I asked myself, what if I could combine two of my favorite things: avocados and hummus into something like a guacamole hummus? Would the sky fall? Would my taste buds explode? And so, this recipe was born.

MIND foods: Beans, olive oil, fruits

Yield: 4 to 6 servings

Prep time: 15 minutes

1 (15-ounce) can of low-sodium chickpeas, drained and rinsed

3 tablespoons olive oil

1½ tablespoon tahini

1 lime, juiced

1 clove garlic, peeled

⅛ teaspoon ground cumin

2 medium ripe avocados

handful finely chopped cilantro leaves

black pepper, to taste

crushed red pepper flakes, to taste

1. In a food processor, pulse chickpeas, olive oil, tahini, lime juice, and garlic until smooth.

2. Season with pepper to taste, add cumin and avocados, and pulse mixture until smooth.

3. Sprinkle with cilantro and crushed red pepper flakes to taste. Serve with fresh vegetables or low-sodium tortilla chips.

BEET HUMMUS

I make this beet hummus whenever we have company over because this dish is not only delicious and healthy, but the garnish is such a nice added touch. It's always a hit because people love its presentation and, of course, how yummy it is.

MIND foods: Vegetables, beans, olive oil

Yield: 4 to 6 servings

Prep time: 15 minutes   **Cook time:** 45 minutes

1 medium beet, greens still attached

¼ cup water

1 (15-ounce) can chickpeas, well drained and rinsed

2 cloves garlic, minced

3 tablespoons tahini

1 lemon, juiced

pinch lemon zest

1 teaspoon ground cumin

½ teaspoon ground coriander

¼ cup extra-virgin olive oil

1 tablespoon grapeseed oil (optional)

1. Preheat the oven to 400°F.

2. Slice the beet greens off and set to the side. In a small deep baking dish, add the beet, along with the ¼ cup of water. Cover the baking dish and transfer to the oven to roast for 45 minutes, until the beet is tender. Let the beet cool, and make sure to save the beet juice.

3. Slice off the top of the beet, peel off the outer layer, and cut the beet into cubes.

4. In a blender or food processor, add the beet, chickpeas, garlic, tahini, lemon juice, lemon zest, ground cumin, ground coriander, olive oil, and a splash of beet juice, and blend until smooth. Add beet juice as necessary for desired consistency. Remove when hummus reaches desired texture.

5. To make a garnish with the beet green, heat a tablespoon of grapeseed oil over medium-high heat in a skillet. Slice up the beet greens and discard the stem. Sprinkle the beet greens with a bit of cumin, coriander, and a touch of salt, and add them to the skillet. Sauté until pan fried.

6. Remove from heat and let cool. When cool, break up the fried beet greens into small pieces and garnish the beet hummus.

VEGAN PARMESAN "CHEESE"

A better option for the MIND Diet is, of course, nondairy cheese. This cashew cheese option has the texture and flavor of Parmesan but the health benefits of cashews. Enjoy on your favorite pasta dish.

MIND food: Nuts
Yield: 4 to 6 servings
Prep time: 5 minutes

1 cup raw cashews

¼ cup nutritional yeast

½ teaspoon garlic powder

salt and pepper, to taste

Put the ingredients in a food processor or high speed blender and pulse until a fine, sprinkly texture is achieved.

PIZZA SAUCE

Sure, you can use sauce from a jar, but why would you? This recipe is super easy to make and delicious.

MIND food: Vegetables

Yield: 8 to 10 servings

Prep time: 5 minutes   **Cook time:** 25 minutes

1 tablespoon grapeseed oil	1 tablespoon honey
¼ medium sweet yellow onion	½ teaspoon dried basil
	½ teaspoon dried oregano
2 cloves garlic, minced	¼ teaspoon salt
1 (15-ounce) can low-sodium tomato sauce	

1. Heat 1 tablespoon of grapeseed oil in a large skillet over medium heat. Add onion and garlic.

2. Cook for 5 minutes, stirring often. Remove from heat and set aside, draining any extra liquid.

3. In a bowl, combine tomato sauce, honey, basil, oregano, and salt.

4. Combine all ingredients in a medium sauce pot. Cook, over medium low heat, for 15 to 20 minutes, stirring occasionally.

5. Spread over prepared pizza dough and bake, or store, refrigerated for up to 1 week, in an airtight container until ready to cook.

WHOLE GRAIN PIZZA DOUGH

It's important to eat whole grains rather than refined grains, because refined grains are stripped of their valuable nutrients during the refining process. This recipe retains that whole-grain goodness, and includes B vitamins, fiber, iron, and omega-3s. Plus, it's fun to knead your own dough—a great activity to do alone, as a couple, or for a family.

MIND foods: Whole grains, olive oil, nuts

Yield: 8 to 10 servings

Prep time: 3 hours   **Cook time:** 10 minutes

2 tablespoons whole-grain bulgur wheat	1½ cups whole wheat flour, plus more for kneading
2 tablespoons quinoa	dash salt
¾ cup warm water	1 tablespoon olive oil
1 teaspoon honey	1 tablespoon ground flax seeds
1 teaspoon active dry yeast	1 tablespoon sunflower seeds

1. Bring 2 cups of water to a boil in a small pot. Add the bulgur wheat and quinoa and cook for 10 minutes. Remove from heat and place grains in a fine meshed strainer and run under cold water to stop their cooking. Set them aside to drain in the strainer for 10 to 15 minutes.

2. On a thick layer of paper towels, spread the grains out in an even layer. Gently pat the top with more paper towels to absorb any extra moisture.

3. Stir together the warm water, honey, and yeast in a small bowl. Let the mixture sit until a small layer of foam forms at the top, 3 to 5 minutes.

4. Combine the whole wheat flour and a dash of salt in a large bowl. Then add the yeast mixture and olive oil and mix together with a rubber spatula.

5. When you can see the dough starting to take shape, mix in the grains that have been drying on the paper towels. Add the flax seeds and the sunflower seeds.

6. Form the dough into a ball in the center of the bowl, scraping the sides for any extra. Cover the bowl with plastic wrap and keep in a warm (but not hot) place until the dough has doubled in size, about 2 hours.

7. After the dough has doubled, dust a baking sheet with flour. Sprinkle more flour on a clean, dry work surface and add some flour onto your hands to prevent sticking. Scrape the dough onto the floured surface and knead gently for a couple of minutes, adding in just enough flour to make the dough less sticky but still moist. Don't let it get too dry.

8. Form the dough into 1 ball for 1 pizza, or divide it into smaller balls for little pizzas. Place the dough ball(s) on the prepared baking sheet. Cover loosely with plastic wrap let it rest for 30 minutes.

9. After 30 minutes, the dough can be shaped into crusts and cooked as desired, or left in ball form and stored, covered, in the refrigerator, for up to 2 weeks.

HOMEMADE HONEY-ROASTED VANILLA BEAN ALMOND BUTTER

Almond butter is sweet, salty, and delicious. Almond butter is slightly sweeter than peanut butter, and is also easier for the body to digest. Almonds contain zinc, a mineral that helps fight free radicals that cause oxidative stress. They're also loaded with vitamins and nutrients like vitamin E, vitamin B6, and omega-3s. Vanilla bean also contains minerals like potassium, magnesium, and manganese. Keep this recipe a little crunchy or blend it until smooth, and enjoy it on sandwiches, on crackers, or right on your spoon. For a revamped classic, try this on whole grain bread with fruit spread or local honey for an AB & J.

Mind food: Nuts

Yield: 16 servings

Prep time: 25 minutes   **Cook time:** 15 minutes

2 cups unsalted almonds

dash sea salt

1 vanilla bean, split lengthwise and seeds scraped

1 teaspoon local honey

1. Preheat oven to 350°F.

2. Spread almonds evenly on a baking sheet and roast in the oven for 12 to 15 minutes or until slightly brown. Be careful not to burn.

3. Carefully transfer the almonds to your food processor or high speed blender and process for 10 to 15 minutes, scraping down the sides often. The almonds should start to clump together. Continue to process until you reach your desired texture.

4. Add the salt, vanilla bean, and honey, and process for another minute or so until blended.

5. Store in an airtight container, refrigerated, for up to 2 weeks. Stir before use to combine the oils.

LOW-SODIUM BLACKENING SEASONING

A great way to change up your fish or chicken is to serve it blackened. One of my dad's favorite dishes is blackened salmon, and I always try to make it for him when we visit. This seasoning is low in sodium and is easy and quick to make. If stored properly, it lasts just as long as what you'd buy in the store.

Yield: 12 to 14 servings

Prep time: 5 minutes

1½ tablespoons ground paprika

1 tablespoon garlic powder

1 tablespoon onion powder

1 tablespoon dried thyme

1 teaspoon black pepper

1 teaspoon cayenne pepper

1 teaspoon dried basil

1 teaspoon dried oregano

Combine all ingredients well and store in an airtight container or jar.

MANGO GUACAMOLE

Mangoes are a delicious, high-fiber fruit full of vitamin A, vitamin C, B vitamins, potassium, and even copper. For this recipe, use more or less jalapeño to adjust the spice levels.

MIND food: Fruits

Yield: 6 servings

Prep time: 15 minutes

3 avocados, pits removed

¼ cup red onion, diced

1 jalapeño, seeded and diced

¼ cup chopped fresh cilantro, plus extra for garnish

1 small lime, juiced

1 mango, peeled, diced, pit removed

salt and pepper, to taste

In a medium bowl, mash the avocado. Add the diced red onion, jalapeño, cilantro, lime juice, and mango. Stir gently to combine, then add salt and pepper to taste. Garnish with remaining cilantro.

LEMON VINAIGRETTE

This bright, lemony dressing pairs well with fresh summer salads with lettuces like arugula, romaine, and mixed greens. The polyphenols found in olive oil are strong antioxidants that have been shown to help promote brain health, and even reverse learning and memory deficits.

MIND foods: Olive oil, vegetables

Yield: 6 servings

Prep time: 5 minutes

½ cup olive oil	1 tablespoon local honey
1 lemon, juiced	1 teaspoon dried basil
2 cloves garlic, minced	salt and pepper, to taste

In a small bowl or jar, whisk together ingredients until smooth and well combined. Season with salt and pepper to taste.

CHAPTER 7

DESSERTS

Dessert is one of life's simple pleasures. As we know, dessert and treats aren't something we should enjoy all of the time, but we can still get some benefits out of them when we do. In this chapter, you will find desserts that can be healthy and provide nutritional benefits. Instead of reaching for processed sweets or treats, make one of these.

The recipes here vary, but they all have some benefit built in, and none of them sacrifice on taste.

Mind–Body Tip: Are you up to date on the latest news? Check out the newspaper—local, national, global. What's going on in your world? Learning about the news of the world around us helps keep our brains sharp.

NANNY'S BANANA BREAD

Whole wheat flour, light cream cheese, and maple syrup help make this classic MIND Diet–friendly. You can freeze old bananas for this recipe instead of waiting for new ones to ripen.

MIND foods: Whole grains, berries

Yield: 12 servings

Prep time: 20 minutes   **Cook time:** 1 hour

cooking spray

1⅔ cups whole wheat flour

1 teaspoon baking soda

¼ teaspoon cinnamon

dash salt

1 cup plus 2 tablespoons turbinado sugar

2 eggs

½ cup grapeseed oil

4 very ripe bananas, peeled and mashed

2 tablespoons light cream cheese

1 teaspoon maple syrup

1 cup blueberries, tossed in 1 tablespoon whole wheat flour, or chocolate chips (optional)

1. Preheat oven to 350°F. Grease 2 loaf pans with cooking spray.

2. Sift together the flour, baking soda, cinnamon, and salt in a large bowl and set aside.

3. In a stand mixer or large mixing bowl, beat together sugar and eggs until light and fluffy. Add the oil and gently mix.

4. Add the bananas, cream cheese, and maple syrup to the stand mixer and gently mix, but don't over beat.

4. Slowly sift in the dry ingredient mixture and combine until just incorporated.

5. Add the blueberries or chocolate chips, if desired, and stir to incorporate.

6. Pour the combined mixture evenly into loaf pans and bake for 45 minutes to 1 hour or until a toothpick inserted in center comes out clean. Remove and let cool.

EGG- AND DAIRY-FREE GINGERBREAD COOKIES

By eliminating eggs and dairy from these cookies, we eliminate saturated fats that may reduce cognitive functioning and cause inflammation. This is why we stick to low-fat dairy, like low-fat cheese, when necessary, on the MIND Diet, or find a nondairy alternative. These cookies are crispy and spicy—enjoy them any time of year.

MIND food: Whole grains

Yield: 16 to 20 servings

Prep time: 2 hours **Cook time:** 8 to 9 minutes

2 cups whole wheat flour plus extra, as needed

½ teaspoon baking soda

½ teaspoon baking powder

1½ teaspoons ground ginger

½ teaspoon ground nutmeg

½ teaspoon ground cinnamon

½ teaspoon ground cloves

dash salt

⅓ cup butter

¾ cup turbinado sugar

¼ cup molasses

¼ cup unsweetened nondairy milk

cooking spray

1. Combine the flour, baking soda, baking powder, ginger, nutmeg, cinnamon, cloves and salt in a medium bowl and set aside.

2. In a stand mixer or large mixing bowl, beat the butter and sugar until light and fluffy. Add the molasses and milk and combine.

3. Slowly add the dry ingredients to the wet mixture until a stiff dough forms. Flatten it into a disc, wrap in plastic wrap, and refrigerate for at least 1 hour.

4. Preheat the oven to 350°F. Grease a baking tray with cooking spray.

5. On a flat, clean surface, sift out a few tablespoons of flour and flour your hands. Roll out the dough to ¼-inch thick. Cut into shapes. Bake for 8 to 9 minutes.

6. Remove and let cool.

GREEK YOGURT HONEY SAUCE

This recipe is so light and sweet, it's perfect for hot summer days and late afternoon picnics. Whenever someone asks you to bring dessert to a picnic, let this be your go-to. Serve with fresh fruit or granola.

Mind food: Fruits

Yield: 6 to 8 servings

Prep time: 5 minutes

2 cups low-fat Greek yogurt

½ cup local honey

1 teaspoon vanilla extract

¼ teaspoon ground cinnamon

1 banana, sliced

1 mango, pit removed, chopped

1 cup blueberries

1 cup strawberries, sliced

1 cup raspberries

1. Combine the yogurt, honey, vanilla, and cinnamon in a bowl and stir together.

2. Mix the fruit together in a bowl. Pour the yogurt mixture over the fruit.

CHICKY BLONDIES

I'm normally not a fan of beans in desserts. These blondies, however, are the perfect combination of light, sweet flavors. The chickpeas add texture and flavor, instead of tasting like a mouthful of beans. These are great for introducing your family to vegetable-friendly options. Whether you tell them before or after they taste these treats is up to you. Try making these with the Honey-Roasted Vanilla Bean Almond Butter (page 174).

MIND foods: Beans, nuts

Yield: 12 servings

Prep time: 10 minutes   **Cook time:** 25 minutes

cooking spray

1 (15-ounce) can no-sodium chickpeas, rinsed and drained

½ cup Homemade Honey-Roasted Vanilla Bean Almond Butter (page 174) or peanut butter

⅓ cup pure maple syrup or local honey

2 teaspoons vanilla extract

½ teaspoon salt

¼ teaspoon baking powder

¼ teaspoon baking soda

¼ cup chocolate chips plus 2 tablespoons

1. Preheat oven to 350°F and grease an 8x8-inch baking pan with cooking spray.

2. In a food processor or high speed blender, combine all ingredients except chocolate chips and process until smooth.

3. Fold ⅓ cup of chocolate chips into the batter.

4. Spread batter evenly in the prepared pan, then sprinkle 2 tablespoons of chocolate chips on top.

5. Bake for 20 to 25 minutes or until the edges are golden brown and the center is firm.

6. Remove from oven and let cool.

SUMMER FRUIT POPS

Is there anything more refreshing, and nostalgic, than a fruit pop on a summer day? Red and purple were my favorite "flavors" when I was growing up. These easy-to-make alternatives are all natural, MIND Diet–friendly, fun to make, and super refreshing. You can use ice pop molds for these, but any non-stick 5- to 6-ounce cup that you can use as a makeshift ice pop mold will do. Or, make them as frozen treat cups!

MIND foods: Berries, fruits

Yield: 8 servings

Prep time: 10 minutes **Freezing time:** 4 to 6 hours

2 kiwis, peeled and sliced into ¼-inch slices

½ cup blueberries

1 cup diced strawberries

1 cup fresh pineapple or orange juice

1. Toss and mix the diced fruit in a medium-sized bowl. Fill each ice pop mold or cup with fruit. Add 1 tablespoon of juice into each mold or cup, and if using a mold, insert ice pop sticks.

2. Freeze until firm. To remove the ice pops from the molds or cups, run the bases under warm water for a few seconds and gently wiggle the pops out.

ROASTED PEARS WITH CHOPPED WALNUTS

This recipe is classy and perfect to serve for company when you don't have a lot of time. I make this when we have last minute guests and I only have time to quickly shop.

MIND food: Nuts

Yield: 4 servings

Prep time: 5 minutes   **Cook time:** 30 minutes

4 large ripe pears	½ teaspoon ground cinnamon
4 teaspoons local honey	½ cup walnuts, chopped finely

1. Preheat the oven to 350°F.

2. Cut the pears in half lengthwise and remove the seeds and stems. Place them on a baking sheet.

3. Drizzle each pear half with ½ teaspoon of honey and then sprinkle with cinnamon. Top the halves with chopped walnuts.

4. Bake the pears for 30 minutes. Finish under the broiler for 30 seconds to a minute for extra crunchy walnuts and a lovely caramelization.

CHOCOLATE BOURBON PECAN PIE

When I moved to the South, I discovered the joy of pecan pie: It comes in so many varieties, there's an option for everyone. This one, which includes chocolate and bourbon, is sweet, crunchy, and of course, bourbon-y. What more could you want from dessert?

MIND foods: Whole grains, nuts

Yield: 10 to 12 servings

Prep time: 30 minutes   **Cook time:** 50 minutes

1 whole wheat pie crust	½ cup brown sugar
2 cups raw pecan halves or pieces	1 tablespoon bourbon or amaretto (optional)
1 cup maple syrup	1 teaspoon vanilla extract
2 tablespoons butter	dash salt
3 large eggs	½ cup dark chocolate chips

1. Preheat the oven to 375°F.

2. Spread the crust into a pie plate. Bake for 3 to 5 minutes, to set the crust. Use pie weights if you have them to keep the crust from bubbling, but if not, a little bubbly crust never hurt anyone.

3. Remove the crust from the oven and set aside.

4. In a medium pan, toast the pecans over medium heat for 3 to 5 minutes, or until just lightly toasted. Remove from heat and set aside.

5. In a small pot, combine the maple syrup and butter over medium-low heat. Cook, stirring occasionally, until the butter melts for about 30 seconds. Remove from heat.

6. In a stand mixer or large bowl, whisk the eggs and then whisk in the brown sugar, bourbon or amaretto (if desired), vanilla, and salt.

7. Gradually add the maple syrup mixture into the egg mixture, stirring to combine. Fold in the pecans. Finally, fold in the chocolate chips.

8. Pour the pecan mixture into the prepared pie crust and bake for 30 to 40 minutes, or until the center of the pie is no longer liquid. Remove from the oven and allow to cool completely before serving.

HOMESTYLE APPLE PIE

The whole wheat crust and local honey in this recipe, help make this classic dish MIND-Diet–friendly. Cinnamon, used here as a mild spice, may also help delay or reverse cognitive impairment.

MIND food: Whole grains

Yield: 10 to 12 servings

Prep time: 20 minutes   **Cook time:** 50 minutes

2 whole wheat pie crusts

4 Granny Smith apples, peeled, cored, and chopped

4 Honey Crisp or Macintosh apples, peeled, cored, and chopped

1 teaspoon ground cinnamon

¾ cup local honey

2 tablespoons butter

2 tablespoons whole wheat flour

1. Preheat the oven to 450°F.

2. Spread 1 of the crusts into a pie plate. Bake for 3 to 5 minutes to set the crust. Use pie weights if you have them to keep the crust from bubbling, but if not, a little bubbly crust never hurt anyone. Remove from the oven and set aside.

3. In a large bowl, combine the apples, cinnamon, and honey. Stir well to coat evenly.

4. Pour the mixture into the prepared crust. Dot evenly with the butter. Sprinkle with whole wheat flour.

5. Cover with the other pie crust and press the edges together, sealing them. Using a fork, poke several holes in the top of the crust.

6. Bake at 450°F for 15 minutes and then reduce heat to 350°F and bake for 30 to 35 minutes, until apples are tender. Remove and let cool.

OATMEAL COOKIES

Oatmeal provides a flavor, texture, and, of course, nutritional benefit that plain old cookies lack. These are chewy and crunchy and sweet—perfect to have on hand for a full fiber, yummy treat.

MIND food: Whole grains

Yield: 24 servings

Prep time: 20 minutes   **Cook time:** 10 minutes

cooking spray	¾ cup local honey
2 cups whole wheat flour	1½ tablespoons maple syrup
dash salt	2 eggs
½ teaspoon cinnamon	1 tablespoon vanilla extract
1 teaspoon baking powder	1 cup chocolate chips or raisins
1 teaspoon baking soda	
3 cups steel cut oats	3 tablespoons unsweetened nondairy milk
1 cup butter, melted	

1. Preheat the oven to 350°F and spray a baking sheet with cooking spray.

2. Combine the flour, salt, cinnamon, baking powder, baking soda, and oats in a large bowl.

3. In a large bowl or stand mixer, cream together the butter, honey, and maple syrup. Add the eggs, milk, and vanilla and beat until creamy, about 30 seconds.

4. Slowly add the dry ingredients to the wet ingredients and stir to combine. Fold in chocolate chips or raisins.

5. Using a teaspoon, drop the dough onto the prepared baking sheet into small balls. Bake for 8 to 10 minutes or until cooked. Remove and allow to cool.

BAKED PLANTAINS

A plantain, a type of the banana, is usually eaten cooked. I was pleasantly surprised the first time I tried plantains as maduros, or fried plantains. Full of potassium, vitamin A, vitamin C, and B6, these are baked, but you still get the same sweet taste.

MIND food: Berries

Yield: 4 servings

Prep time: 5 minutes   **Cook time:** 15 minutes

cooking spray

4 very ripe plantains, peeled and sliced into quarters

1 tablespoon grapeseed oil

sea salt, to taste

1. Preheat the oven to 450°F.

2. Lightly coat a baking dish with cooking spray.

3. Place the plantains in a single layer in the baking dish and drizzle with oil.

4. Bake for 10 to 15 minutes, until plantains are browned and tender. Remove from the oven and sprinkle with salt.

EASY FRUIT SALAD

What could be more simple than a refreshing fruit salad? This recipe combines some of my favorite summer fruits and adds a little bit of mint for a tinge more color and flavor at the end. This is a great, easy picnic dish. Serve plain or with Greek Yogurt Honey Sauce (page 182).

MIND foods: Berries, fruit

Yield: 8 to 10 servings

Prep time: 20 minutes

4 cups chopped pineapple

1 quart halved strawberries

1 cup seedless green grapes

1 cup seedless red grapes

2 mangoes, peeled, cored, and sliced into chunks

4 kiwis, peeled and sliced into chunks

1 pint raspberries

1 pint blueberries

2 tablespoons chopped fresh mint

Wash all of the produce thoroughly and gently pat it dry or allow to drain. Combine in a large bowl and gently mix together. Sprinkle with mint.

CHAPTER 8
SNACKS

I love to snack, and I've found that my productivity suffers when I deny myself a snack. Grazing can be beneficial to help us maintain a steady blood sugar level—but of course, you have to eat the right kind of snack. We need good nutrition to keep our brains focused and productive throughout the day, as well as to help maintain our memory function. Try out some of my favorite snacks, included here. They're full of healthy fats, protein, and fiber. I bring them to my office or enjoy them when I'm home, reading a good book. Snack away, guilt-free.

Mind–Body Tip: Join a social group. It could be a walking group, a knitting group, or a yoga class; anything where you are meeting with others who have a shared interest or passion. Our social support systems are an important part of keeping our brains healthy.

HUMMUS AND PITA

This is a quick and easy dish that requires almost no prep time if you make the hummus ahead. Not only are chickpeas, used in the hummus, high in fiber, they are also a great source of magnesium, which helps the brain transmit messages and relaxes blood vessels, promoting better blood flow to the brain.

MIND foods: Whole grains, vegetables, olive oil

Yield: 4 servings

Prep time: 5 minutes   **Cook time:** 10 minutes

4 whole wheat pita pockets, cut into triangles

1 tablespoon olive oil

½ teaspoon garlic powder

1 recipe Avocado or Beet Hummus (page 167 or page 168)

1. Preheat the oven to 400°F.

2. Place the pita triangles on a large baking sheet and drizzle with oil. Season with garlic powder. Bake for 8 to 10 minutes, or until pitas are browned.

3. Serve with hummus of your choice.

SNACKY CHICKPEAS

Instead of reaching for chips or crackers, reach for snacky chickpeas, which are high in fiber and brain-healthy vitamins and minerals like B6 and magnesium. I like the flavor of smoked paprika, but you can substitute it for another seasoning or spice that you prefer.

MIND foods: Beans, olive oil

Yield: 4 servings

Prep time: 5 minutes   **Cook time:** 45 minutes

1 (15-ounce) can low- or no-sodium chickpeas, drained and rinsed

½ teaspoon smoked paprika

1 teaspoon olive oil

1. Pat the chickpeas until very dry.

2. Preheat the oven to 350°F. Mix all the ingredients together in a bowl, then spread the chickpeas evenly on a baking sheet. Bake in the oven for 45 minutes or until crunchy.

3. Remove from the oven and let cool.

SWEET AND SPICY NUTS

I often bring this mixture to work for a healthy snack, but it can also be something that you set out for guests to snack on as a pre-dinner appetizer.

MIND food: Nuts

Yield: 10 servings

Prep time: 10 minutes   **Cook time:** 25 minutes

cooking spray or grapeseed oil	⅓ cup maple syrup
3 cups raw cashews	¼ cup brown sugar, lightly packed
2 cups raw walnuts	½ orange, juiced
2 cups raw pecans	2 teaspoons chipotle powder
½ cup raw almonds	2 teaspoons sea salt, divided

1. Preheat the oven to 350°F. Spray a baking pan with cooking spray, or grease the pan lightly with grapeseed oil.

2. In a large bowl, combine the nuts. Add the maple syrup, brown sugar, orange juice, and chipotle powder, and toss well to combine.

3. Spread the nuts, now coated, in an even layer on the pan. Sprinkle with half of the sea salt.

4. Bake for 25 minutes, stirring twice, or until the nuts are browned. Remove from the oven and sprinkle with the remaining salt. Stir to combine.

5. Let the nuts cool at room temperature, stirring occasionally to prevent sticking. Store in an airtight container.

BRUSCHETTA

This combination of flavors is one of my favorites: the fresh acidity of the tomatoes, the tangy vinegar, and the bright basil. This works well as a snack just for you, or to share with guests. Serve plain, or with whole grain crackers, or whole grain toast.

MIND foods: Vegetables, olive oil

Yield: 2 servings

Prep time: 10 minutes

2 tomatoes, sliced

¼ cup vegan or low-fat mozzarella cheese, shredded

1 tablespoon olive oil

1 tablespoon balsamic vinegar

1 tablespoon fresh basil

salt and pepper, to taste

Sprinkle mozzarella onto tomato slices. Drizzle with olive oil and balsamic vinegar. Season with basil, salt, and pepper.

ALT-ANTS ON A LOG

Did your mom make you ants on a log? This version uses any of the hummus recipes you like in this book, plus some yummy olives, to be the "ants." It's crunchy, satisfying, and full of fiber.

MIND foods: Vegetables, beans

Yield: 2 servings

Prep time: 5 minutes

6 celery stalks, cut in half

¼ cup plus 2 tablespoons hummus

¼ cup Kalamata olives, chopped

Spread hummus in cavities of celery stalks. Top with chopped olives. Serve.

TRAIL MIX

I love to snack on trail mix, but when I buy the pre-made versions, there's always at least one addition that I end up avoiding, all the way at the bottom of the bag. Make your own at home, and use any combination of nuts and fruit that you like—just be sure to use more healthy nuts than sweet additions.

MIND food: Nuts

Yield: 6 to 8 servings

Prep time: 5 minutes

½ cup roasted unsalted almonds

½ cup raw walnuts, chopped

¼ cup naturally sweetened or low-sugar raisins

¼ naturally sweetened or low-sugar dried cranberries

2 tablespoons dark chocolate chips

Combine all ingredients and stir together. Store in an airtight container.

CONVERSIONS

VOLUME CONVERSIONS		
U.S.	U.S. EQUIVALENT	METRIC
1 tablespoon (3 teaspoons)	½ fluid ounce	15 milliliters
¼ cup	2 fluid ounces	60 milliliters
⅓ cup	3 fluid ounces	90 milliliters
½ cup	4 fluid ounces	120 milliliters
⅔ cup	5 fluid ounces	150 milliliters
¾ cup	6 fluid ounces	180 milliliters
1 cup	8 fluid ounces	240 milliliters
2 cups	16 fluid ounces	480 milliliters

TEMPERATURE CONVERSIONS	
FAHRENHEIT (°F)	CELSIUS (°C)
125°F	50°C
150°F	65°C
175°F	80°C
200°F	95°C
225°F	110°C
250°F	120°C
275°F	135°C
300°F	150°C
325°F	165°C
350°F	175°C
375°F	190°C
400°F	200°C
425°F	220°C
450°F	230°C

WEIGHT CONVERSIONS	
U.S.	METRIC
½ ounce	15 grams
1 ounce	30 grams
2 ounces	60 grams
¼ pound	115 grams
⅓ pound	150 grams
½ pound	225 grams
¾ pound	350 grams
1 pound	450 grams

RECIPE INDEX

ACKNOWLEDGMENTS

Many thanks to my tireless and fantastic editors, Bridget Thoreson, Alice Riegert, Claire Chun, and Shayna Keyles. This book is so much better for your efforts. Bridget, thank you especially for your kindness, professionalism, and availability—from the first email, you have been wonderful. To Ulysses Press, for publishing this work and for all of the good work it does.

To dear Blair, for being my one-man test kitchen as I worked to create and adapt these recipes over months, and patiently stood by as I wrote this book on weekends and over evenings—thank you for cheering me on. You always do. For all the worlds and the words we've created together (and those that exist only for us). For all those yet to come. Let's go home. Monkey.

Thank you to my Nanny, Shirley Douglas, who instilled in me a love of reading and taught me how to bake. Many of my fondest memories are with you.

Many thanks to you, dear reader. Your mind holds many gifts, the most important being, well, you. And that is why it's so important to keep it healthy. I hope you enjoy these MIND Diet recipes on your path to brain-health.

To my community of friends and peers: for your never-ending support, your love, your warmth. Our shared laughs and our shared sorrows. For every time I've asked for a quick read or an edit and you've been there, and for every time I've needed a friend, and I never had to wonder if I'd be left wanting. I am in your debt—and happy to be there. Thank you.

ABOUT THE AUTHOR

Kristin Diversi is a writer, editor, and nutritionist. She became interested in health and wellness after seeing the role they played in the well-being of the people she loved, sparking a lifelong dedication to learning more about the subjects. She achieved her Master of Science in Nutrition and Food Sciences from Montclair State University in 2013, with a focus on working with children who were neo-phobic—or picky eaters. Kristin has worked in the public sector, teaching nutrition education, and as a private nutrition consultant. She is featured regularly in health and wellness publications and believes that wellness is a whole-body effort that everyone can achieve.